Palliative Practices From A–Z for the Bedside Clinician

Second Edition

Editors

Peg Esper, MSN, MSA, RN, AOCN®, APRN-BC
Kim K. Kuebler, MN, RN, APRN-BC

Oncology Nursing Society
Pittsburgh, PA

ONS Publishing Division
Publisher: Leonard Mafrica, MBA, CAE
Director, Commercial Publishing/Technical Publications Editor: Barbara Sigler, RN, MNEd
Production Manager: Lisa M. George, BA
Staff Editor: Amy Nicoletti, BA
Copy Editor: Laura Pinchot, BA
Graphic Designer: Dany Sjoen

Palliative Practices From A–Z for the Bedside Clinician (Second Edition)

Library of Congress Control Number: 2008927303
ISBN 978-1-890504-70-0

Publisher's Note
This book is published by the Oncology Nursing Society (ONS). ONS neither represents nor guarantees that the practices described herein will, if followed, ensure safe and effective patient care. The recommendations contained in this book reflect ONS's judgment regarding the state of general knowledge and practice in the field as of the date of publication. The recommendations may not be appropriate for use in all circumstances. Those who use this book should make their own determinations regarding specific safe and appropriate patient-care practices, taking into account the personnel, equipment, and practices available at the hospital or other facility at which they are located. The editors and publisher cannot be held responsible for any liability incurred as a consequence from the use or application of any of the contents of this book. Figures and tables are used as examples only. They are not meant to be all-inclusive, nor do they represent endorsement of any particular institution by ONS. Mention of specific products and opinions related to those products do not indicate or imply endorsement by ONS. Web sites mentioned are provided for imformation only; the hosts are responsible for their own content and availability.

ONS publications are originally published in English. Publishers wishing to translate ONS publications must contact the ONS Publishing Division about licensing arrangements. ONS publications cannot be translated without obtaining written permission from ONS. (Individual tables and figures that are reprinted or adapted require additional permission from the original source.) Because translations from English may not always be accurate or precise, ONS disclaims any responsibility for inaccuracies in words or meaning that may occur as a result of the translation. Readers relying on precise information should check the original English version.

Printed in the United States of America

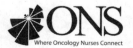

Oncology Nursing Society
Integrity • Innovation • Stewardship • Advocacy • Excellence • Inclusiveness

Contributors

Editors

Peg Esper, MSN, MSA, RN, AOCN®, APRN-BC
Nurse Practitioner, Medical Oncology
University of Michigan
Comprehensive Cancer Center
Ann Arbor, Michigan
Preface; Anorexia, Cachexia, and Nutrition Support; Zoster

Kim K. Kuebler, MN, RN, APRN-BC
Clinical Specialist
Somatic and Neuropathic Pain
The Medical Affairs Company
Savannah, Georgia
Foreword; Preface; Dehydration; Delirium; Appendix C: Internet Resources

Authors

Jerald M. Andry, PharmD, MSc
Clinical Research Associate DRA-MA
Roxane Laboratories, Inc.
Columbus, Ohio
Dyspnea; Hiccups

Catherine Christen, PharmD
Clinical Pharmacist and Clinical
    Assistant Professor
University of Michigan Hospitals and
    College of Pharmacy
Ann Arbor, Michigan
Appendix A: Polypharmacy in Palliative Care

Mellar P. Davis, MD, FCCP
Director of Research
The Harry R. Horvitz Center for
    Palliative Medicine
Cleveland, Ohio
Nausea and Vomiting; Pain

Georgia M. Decker, MS, APRN-BC,
    CN®, AOCN®
Nurse Practitioner
Integrative Care
Albany, New York
Complementary and Alternative Medicine and Integrative Medicine

Suzanne Dixon, MPH, MS, RD
Vice President, Nutrition
P4 Healthcare, LLC
Portland, Oregon
*Anorexia, Cachexia, and Nutrition
Support*

John Travis Dunlap, MSN, ANP-BC
Instructor of Nursing
Vanderbilt University School of
   Nursing
Nashville, Tennessee
Fever

Linda H. Eaton, MN, RN, AOCN®
Research Associate
Oncology Nursing Society
Pittsburgh, Pennsylvania
*Introduction to Evidence-Based
Practice*

Jennifer Fournier, RN, MSN, AOCN®,
   CHPN
Clinical Nurse Specialist
Hospice Savannah, Inc.
Savannah, Georgia
Anxiety; Cough; Fatigue

David Frame, PharmD
Clinical Assistant Professor, Clinical
   Heme/Oncology Specialist
University of Michigan
Ann Arbor, Michigan
*Appendix B: Principles of
Pharmacokinetic Drug Interactions*

Donald L. Garrison, Lic. Funeral
   Director & Emb.
Spring Hill Funeral Home
   and Cemetery
Nashville, Tennessee
Funeral Planning

Ruth Canty Gholz, RN, MS, AOCN®
Oncology Clinical Nurse Specialist
Cincinnati VA Medical Center
Cincinnati, Ohio
Bleeding

Uthona R. Green, RN, MSN
Nurse Manager
Outpatient Clinics
Dayton VA Medical Center
Dayton, Ohio
Urinary Elimination

Debra E. Heidrich, MSN, RN,
   ACHPN®, AOCN®
Palliative Nurse Clinician
Bethesda North Hospital, TriHealth, Inc.
Cincinnati, Ohio
*Ascites; Death and Dying; Diarrhea;
Edema*

Kathryn J. Hill, MSN, BS, MA,
   APRN, NP-C
Nurse Practitioner
Cloverbottom Developmental Center
Nashville, Tennessee
Funeral Planning

LaDonna Hinkle, RN, MSN, OCN®
Staff Nurse, Outpatient Hematology/
   Oncology Clinic
Dayton VA Medical Center
Dayton, Ohio
Mucositis; Xerostomia

George E. Holburn, MSN
Staff Nurse
Transitional Care Unit
Veterans Affairs Tennessee Valley
   Healthcare System-VISN 9
Murfreesboro, Tennessee
Fever

Charles E. Kemp, FNP, FAAN
Senior Lecturer
Baylor University School of Nursing
Dallas, Texas
Cultural Competence

Cheri Mann, RN, MSN, MA
Assistant Professor of Nursing
Crown College
St. Bonifacius, Minnesota
Palliative Care

Joyce A. Marrs, MS, FNP-BC,
    AOCNP®
Nurse Practitioner
Dayton Physicians, Hematology
    and Oncology
Dayton, Ohio
Anemia

Crystal Dea Moore, PhD, MSW, MA
Social Work Program Director
Skidmore College
Saratoga Springs, New York
Advance Directives; Caregiver Issues

Blaire Barnes Morriss, MSN, APRN-
    BC
Nurse Practitioner
The Downtown Clinic for
    the Homeless
Nashville, Tennessee
Sexuality

Mary E. Murphy, RN, MS, AOCN®,
    ACHPN
Director of Clinical Systems, CNS
    Oncology
Hospice of Dayton Inc.
Dayton, Ohio
*Pruritus; Urinary Elimination;
Xerostomia*

Jill R. Nelson, RN, MSN, APRN-BC
Nurse Practitioner, Palliative Care
    Consult Service
Vanderbilt University Medical Center
Nashville, Tennesee
Infection

Marilyn O'Mallon, RN, MSN
Assistant Professor of Nursing
Armstrong Atlantic State University
Savannah, Georgia
Grief and Bereavement

James C. Pace, DSN, RN, MDiv, ANP-
    BC, FAANP
Professor of Nursing and Coordinator,
    ANP—Palliative Care Program
Vanderbilt University School of
    Nursing
Nashville, Tennessee
*Funeral Planning; Infection; Palliative
Care; Seizures; Sexuality*

Kim Anne Pickett, MS, CRNP
Family Nurse Practitioner
Allen County Health Partners
Salud Community Clinic
Tipp City, Ohio
Insomnia

Valarie A. Pompey, MS, APRN-BC,
    AOCNP®
Oncology Nurse Practitioner
Allied Hematology Oncology, LLC
South Bend, Indiana
*Dehydration; Delirium; Palliative
Sedation*

Sheila H. Ridner, PhD, RN, ACNP
Assistant Professor
Vanderbilt University School of
    Nursing
Nashville, Tennessee
Lymphedema

Samuel Gwin Robbins, MSN, RN,
    MTS, ANP-BC
Staff Nurse
Vanderbilt University Medical Center,
    Medical ICU
Nashville, Tennessee
Seizures

Shawn D. Salkow, PharmD
Project Manager, Managed Markets
Boehringer Ingelheim Pharmaceuticals
Ridgefield, Connecticut
Depression

Pamela Spencer, BA, MSN, BSN, FNP
Family Nurse Practitioner (Palliative
    and Gastroenterology Care),
    Adjuvant Nursing Professor
VA Medical Center
Saginaw, Michigan
Bowel Obstruction; Constipation

Catherine J. Stewart, BSN, RN, APN
Graduate Student in Adult Health
    and Palliative Care
Vanderbilt University
Staff Nurse
Alive Hospice
Nashville, Tennessee
Funeral Planning

Linda A. Upchurch, MSN, ANP-BC,
    CHPN
Instructor of Nursing
Georgia Southern University School
    of Nursing
Statesboro, Georgia
Infection

Doreen A. White, BSN, RN, CWOCN
Certified Wound, Ostomy and
    Continence Nurse Consultant
Springfield, Ohio
Skin Lesions

Contents

Foreword

Kim K. Kuebler, MN, RN, APRN-BC

It is the clinician who walks along the path with the patient and his or her family when they receive the diagnosis of a life-limiting malignancy. It is the clinician who listens to the patient when he or she describes the intensity of symptoms and their effect upon the patient's perceived quality of life. It is the clinician who acts as a patient advocate when reporting patient assessments to the healthcare team and ensuring that appropriate interventions will be initiated into the patient's plan of care. It is the clinician who recognizes the value and importance of applying current evidence-based practice interventions into the management of advanced illness and influencing positive patient-centered outcomes.

Bedside clinicians who provide palliative care require the best evidence to support the skills and knowledge necessary to effectively manage multiple symptoms, address psychological and spiritual issues of patients and families, and help patients to make important healthcare decisions when facing advanced illness. Clinicians who apply the best evidence into clinical practice ensure optimal quality of life for the patient. When evidence-based assessments and interventions are considered thoughtfully by the clinician and combined with the goals of the patient and his or her family, clinical decision making should promote desired patient outcomes (Rutledge & Kuebler, 2005).

The lack of evidence-based care provided to patients with palliative care needs has been well documented over the past decade, and several initiatives have arisen from this burgeoning need. For the first time in history, Americans are living longer and, with a predicted increase in the number of malignancies, will require clinicians skilled in palliative management.

Use of psychometrically sound assessment tools to evaluate specific symptoms and the integration of selected interventions that have been trialed successfully and evaluated effectively promote positive patient outcomes. Understanding specific disease pathophysiology and ensuring the appropriate interventions are used to enable effective metabolism are key to optimal palliative symptom management.

Effective palliative management does not occur from a "cookbook" approach but rather from a patient-specific approach that requires ongoing evaluation of specific disease, concomitant diseases, organ function, metabolism capacity, substance history, psychosocial support systems, and patient participation in his or her plan of care. The clinician can facilitate the conduit of care between the healthcare system and the patient. The clinician is able to hold the lantern, casting light along the trajectory of disease that will allow the patient and family to "live until they die" (Saunders & Baines, 1984, p. 10).

The editors of this second edition have enlisted leaders and experts in the field of palliative care to provide the most current evidence to consider when integrating specific interventions into the patient's plan of care. Understanding the evidence is always important, but more importantly, clinicians must recognize that each patient is unique and that not all interventions effectively work from one patient to another. Through sequential trials of interventions and dosing, the clinician, together with the healthcare team, will discover the best patient results.

References

Rutledge, D.N., & Kuebler, K.K. (2005). Applying evidence to palliative care. *Seminars in Oncology Nursing, 21*, 36–43.

Saunders, C., & Baines, M. (1984). *Living with dying: The management of terminal disease.* Oxford, UK: Oxford University Press.

Preface

In considering compiling a second edition of this text, we needed to feel that something more could be added than just a couple of new interventions and updated references. No doubt was in our minds that *Palliative Practices From A–Z for the Bedside Clinician* filled a void in the palliative care literature. So, keeping the information in this book current was important. As we looked for the "something more" that was needed, we realized that *Professional Competencies* detailed in the first edition was better substituted by taking a hard look at the evidence from which we describe competent practice. The idea of adding the *Level of Evidence* for those sections that offer management strategies made us believe that we could offer something really valuable in a second edition of this book. We hope that you will find that your own practice is strengthened by using evidence to determine practice. Although palliative care has only begun to jump on the evidence-based bandwagon, use of best evidence interventions is of utmost importance to the recipients of palliative care—our patients.

Peg Esper
Kim K. Kuebler

Acknowledgments

I want to acknowledge June Huber for being a wonderful "Grandma June" to my children—you are a blessing! I also acknowledge Bruce Redman, DO, who, in our collaborative practice for many years, has always believed that there is never a time when there is "nothing we can do" for a patient. I thank my wonderful husband, Jerry, for his patience and encouragement with all my projects; and my children, Melissa and Tim, for their love and support.—P.E.

I want to acknowledge my friend and colleague James K. Haveman Jr., former Director of the Michigan Department of Community Health, recent Health Minister to Iraq, and an important advocate for palliative and end-of-life care initiatives nationally and internationally. His work in this field and his recognition of the valuable role that the clinician has for the patient living and dying from advanced illness does not go unnoticed.—K.K.

The editors would like to acknowledge the memories of Donald Spencer and Ross Evan Breitbart—husband and nephew to our invited authors—whose deaths arrived at an untimely hour of sudden loss during the development of this textbook.

Introduction to Evidence-Based Practice

Linda H. Eaton, MN, RN, AOCN®

Evidence-based practice is the integration of the best research evidence with clinical expertise and patient values to facilitate clinical decision making (DiCenso, Guyatt, & Ciliska, 2005). The highest quality of care is given to patients and their families when clinicians integrate the critical appraisal of the evidence, their own clinical expertise and experiences, and patient preferences and values when making a practice decision or practice change. Clinical practice that is based upon the best evidence can reduce the uncertainty that patients, families, and healthcare professionals may experience in a complex healthcare system (Melnyk & Fineout-Overholt, 2005).

The concept of evidence-based practice is not new to nursing; since the early 1980s, it has gained momentum and is used to identify and validate even the most basic nursing care procedures (Domrose, 2001). Nursing interventions based on the best evidence are essential for improving patient outcomes.

Evidence-Based Practice Process

Evidence-based practice is a multistep process (Melnyk & Fineout-Overholt, 2005; Oncology Nursing Society [ONS], 2007) and includes the following.
- Identifying a clinical question or problem
- Finding the most relevant and best evidence
- Critically appraising the evidence
- Integrating the evidence with one's clinical expertise, patient preferences, and values in recommending a practice change
- Implementing the practice change
- Evaluating the practice change

Identifying a clinical question or problem that is well developed is critical for conducting an effective search in finding the most relevant and best evidence. The clinical question should identify the patient population (P), a specific intervention (I) of interest, a comparison (C) intervention, and a patient outcome (O). These components are known as the PICO format (Melnyk & Fineout-Overholt, 2005). An example of a PICO question in addressing palliative care is in patients with metastatic lung cancer (P), how effective are opioid analgesics (I) versus acupuncture (C) in the relief of neuropathic pain (O)?

The best evidence refers to methodologically sound, clinically relevant research (DiCenso et al., 2005). The strongest type of evidence comes from systematic reviews, meta-analyses, and evidence-based clinical practice guidelines that are based on findings from randomized controlled trials (Guyatt & Rennie, 2002). A systematic review is a summary of all the research evidence on a particular topic using a rigorous process for searching, retrieving, appraising, and synthesizing studies to answer a specific clinical question. Systematic reviews that incorporate quantitative methods to summarize the results from multiple studies are called meta-analyses. An excellent source for systematic reviews on palliative care is the Cochrane Library of Systematic Reviews, which currently has 43 systematic reviews that address palliative care (Cochrane Collaboration, 2008).

Evidence-based clinical practice guidelines provide practice recommendations developed by a group of experts who perform a methodologically rigorous review of the best evidence on a specific topic (Melnyk & Fineout-Overholt, 2005). Not all clinical practice guidelines are evidence-based because of a paucity of research and may be developed partially or entirely by expert opinion. When considering clinical practice recommendations identified by specific guidelines, the clinician must review the method used in the development of the guidelines.

If systematic reviews, meta-analyses, and evidence-based clinical practice guidelines have not been published, the next type of evidence that should be searched for is randomized controlled trials. If this level of research has not been conducted, the search should continue for other types of studies, such as descriptive or qualitative research (Melnyk & Fineout-Overholt, 2005).

Systematic approaches to assessing the strength of the scientific evidence are available in the literature (Greer, Mosser, Logan, & Halaas, 2000; Guyatt & Rennie, 2002; Melnyk & Fineout-Overholt, 2005; Hadorn, Baker, Hodges, & Hicks, 1996; Harris et al., 2001; Ropka & Spencer-Cisek, 2001; West et al., 2002). Levels of evidence schemas help to prioritize the review and critical appraisal of the research literature because research of stronger study design should be the focus.

The ONS Levels of Evidence schema used within this edition identifies the strength of the research evidence supporting specific interventions in the management of patients living with and dying from advanced malignancy. Level I (high level of evidence) includes systematic reviews and meta-analyses that are based upon well-designed randomized controlled trials; one well-designed randomized controlled trial; and a well-designed trial without randomization. Systematic reviews of nonexperimental design studies, well-conducted case-control studies, poorly controlled studies, consensus reports, and practice guidelines are considered level II (moderate level of evidence). Level III (low level of evidence) is assigned to qualitative designs, case studies, and expert opinion (Ropka & Spencer-Cisek, 2001). This schema is based on the 2001 ONS Priority Symptom Management Project's Levels of Evidence, which was adapted from Hadorn et al.'s (1996) quality rating criteria (Ropka & Spencer Cisek). Understanding the levels of evidence is essential for discerning palliative care interventions to manage specific symptoms in the patient with advanced cancer.

Critically appraising the evidence provides an evaluation of the quality of the research used to address specific clinical questions. Appraisal is essential when critically evaluating the scientific merit and applicability of the evidence to patient care. If the evidence is not critiqued adequately prior to implementing an intervention, specific patient outcomes may be adversely affected (Fain, 2004). Three basic questions are used when critically appraising the research (Ciliska, Cullum, & Marks, 2001; Melnyk & Fineout-Overholt, 2005).

- What are the results of the study?
- Are the results from the study valid?
- Will the results be useful in developing a plan of care for my patients?

Additional guidelines for critiquing research studies are available from other resources, such as nursing research textbooks (Fain, 2004; ONS, 2007).

When recommending a practice change, integrating the evidence with personal clinical expertise and experiences and the patient's preferences and values will increase the likelihood of an effective change. Additional components to consider when making a practice change include healthcare resources and risk-benefit analysis for the individual patient (Melnyk & Fineout-Overholt, 2005; ONS, 2007).

Implementing the practice change at the patient level or at the clinical setting level is the next step in the evidence-based practice process. If the scientific evidence demonstrates that acupuncture is as effective as opioid analgesics in relieving neuropathic pain in patients with metastatic lung cancer and the patient has requested this intervention, this would be a practice change at the patient level. If the practice change is made for all patients with metastatic lung cancer experiencing neuropathic pain in a clinical setting, this would be a practice change at the clinical level. The approval process for implementing a practice change at this level should be determined, in addition to identifying potential barriers and specific facilitators who would advocate for making a practice change at the clinical setting level (ONS, 2007).

Evaluating the practice change is the final step of the evidence-based practice process and is critical in determining whether the practice change resulted in the expected outcomes. If the example of using acupuncture for relieving pain in the patient with metastatic lung cancer did not produce the expected results, then possible explanations for the patient outcomes should be examined (e.g., nonadherence to the acupuncture by the patient, improper technique used, intervention delivered differently in practice than what was described in the research literature, different patient demographics than those of the study sample). Based on the patient outcomes, the intervention is either accepted, rejected, or modified (Goode, 1995).

Evidence-Based Practice and Palliative Care

Palliative care is an evolving specialty that requires the nursing skills and knowledge that come from understanding the current scientific evidence and its application to patients living with and dying from advanced illness. Conducting methodologically rigorous palliative care research is a challenge in this patient population. Although the randomized controlled trial is the gold standard in determining the efficacy of palliative care interventions, clinical research is limited for several reasons. Ethical and moral issues often arise when conducting research with patients who are seriously ill and have a poor prognosis coupled with high attrition rates (Higginson, 1999).

Outcome measures for patients receiving palliative care differ from other patient groups; for example, the primary outcome for most nonpalliative care patients is survival. Quality of life is an appropriate outcome for palliative care patients; however, measuring outcomes such as quality of life, including quality of death, quality of care, and the best resolution of bereavement when patients are seriously ill is difficult (Wilkinson, 1998). Two organizations, the Agency for Healthcare Research and Quality (AHRQ) and the National Quality Forum (NQF), have addressed cancer care quality measures at the end of life. The AHRQ has identified measures for addressing pain, dyspnea, depression, and advance care planning in palliative cancer care, but these measures need to be tested in relevant populations. The NQF has endorsed a standardized set of performance measures to assess the quality of cancer care at the end of life (Lorenz et al., 2006; NQF, 2007).

For the bedside clinician, understanding and appreciating the available scientific evidence is important when selecting specific interventions to improve the overall quality of life for the patient and his or her family. This text provides palliative care practices that are based on current evidence for the management of physical, emotional, and social aspects encountered by the patient living with and dying from advanced illness.

References

Ciliska, D., Cullum, N., & Marks, S. (2001). Evaluation of systematic reviews of treatment or prevention interventions. *Evidence-Based Nursing, 4,* 100–104.

Cochrane Collaboration. (2008). *The Cochrane library of systematic reviews.* Retrieved January 11, 2008, from http://www.mrw.interscience.wiley.com/cochrane

DiCenso, A., Guyatt, G., & Ciliska, D. (2005). *Evidence-based nursing: A guide to clinical practice.* St. Louis, MO: Mosby.

Domrose, C. (2001, November 26). A second look: Traditional methods come under scrutiny as healthcare professionals base more clinical procedures on evidence-based practice. *NurseWeek,* pp. 1–4.

Fain, J.A. (2004). *Reading, understanding, and applying nursing research: A text and workbook* (2nd ed.). Philadelphia: F.A. Davis.

Goode, C.J. (1995). Evaluation of research-based nursing practice. *Nursing Clinics of North America, 30,* 421–428.

Greer, N., Mosser, G., Logan, G., & Halaas, G.W. (2000). A practical approach to evidence grading. *Joint Commission Journal on Quality Improvement, 26,* 700–712.

Guyatt, G., & Rennie, D. (2002). *Users' guides to the medical literature: Essentials of evidence-based clinical practice/The Evidence-Based Medicine Working Group.* Chicago: American Medical Association Press.

Hadorn, D.C., Baker, D., Hodges, J.S., & Hicks, N. (1996). Rating the quality of evidence for clinical practice guidelines. *Journal of Clinical Epidemiology, 49,* 749–754.

Harris, R.P., Hefland, M., Woolf, S.H., Lohr, K.N., Mulrow, C.D., Teutsch, S.M., et al. (2001). Current methods of the U.S. Preventive Services Task Force: A review of the process. *American Journal of Preventive Medicine, 20,* 21–35.

Higginson, I.J. (1999). Evidence-based palliative care: There is some evidence—and there needs to be more. *BMJ, 319,* 462–463.

Lorenz, K., Lynn, K., Dy, S., Hughes, R., Mularski, R., Shugarman, L., et al. (2006). *Cancer care quality measures: Symptoms and end-of-life care.* Evidence Report/Technology Assessment No. 137 (Prepared by the Southern California Evidence-Based Practice Center under Contract No. 290-02-003) [AHRQ Publication No. 06-E001]. Rockville, MD: Agency for Healthcare Research and Quality.

Melnyk, B.M., & Fineout-Overholt, E. (2005). *Evidence-based practice in nursing and healthcare: A guide to best practice.* Philadelphia: Lippincott Williams & Wilkins.

National Quality Forum. (2007). *Quality of cancer care performance measures: Phase II.* Retrieved June 15, 2007, from http://www.qualityforum.org/projects/ongoing/cancer/index.asp

Oncology Nursing Society. (2007). *Evidence-based practice resource area: EBP process.* Retrieved May 25, 2007, from http://www.ons.org/evidence

Ropka, M.E., & Spencer-Cisek, P. (2001). PRISM: Priority symptom management project phase I: Assessment. *Oncology Nursing Forum, 28,* 1585–1594.

West, S., King, V., Carey, T., Lohr, K., McKoy, N., Sutton, S., et al. (2002). *Systems to rate the strength of the evidence* [AHRQ Publication No. 02-3016]. Rockville, MD: Agency for Healthcare Research and Quality.

Wilkinson, S. (1998). The importance of evidence-based care. *International Journal of Palliative Nursing, 4,* 160.

Evidence-Based Practice Resources

- Academic Center for Evidence-Based Practice
  www.acestar.uthscsa.edu/resources_www.htm
- Agency for Healthcare Research and Quality
  www.ahrq.gov
- Centre for Evidence-Based Nursing (York, United Kingdom)
  www.york.ac.uk/healthsciences/centres/evidence/cebn.htm
- Cochrane Collaboration
  www.cochrane.org
- Evidence-Based Medicine Toolkit
  www.ebm.med.ualberta.ca
- German Centre for Evidence-Based Nursing
  http://pflegeforschung.de
- Joanna Briggs Institute
  www.joannabriggs.edu.au
- Oncology Nursing Society Evidence-Based Practice Resource Area
  www.ons.org/evidence
- Sarah Cole Hirsh Institute
  http://fpb.cwru.edu/HirshInstitute
- School of Health and Related Research Netting the Evidence
  www.shef.ac.uk/scharr/ir/netting
- Turning Research Into Practice
  www.tripdatabase.com

Generic Medications and Brand-Name Equivalents

This list is not comprehensive; more than one company may manufacture or market a product by the same name. Although every effort was made to ensure the accuracy of this information at press time, product and company information change frequently; therefore, the publishers and contributors disclaim responsibility for the accuracy of this list. Before using this information, verify it to ensure that it is up to date. Cited trademark status pertains to the United States only. All products listed may not be available in the United States. This list is not an assertion of trademark ownership or an endorsement of any product.

Acyclovir, Zovirax®, GlaxoSmithKline

Albuterol, Proventil®, Schering-Plough

Allopurinol, Zyloprim®, Prometheus Labs

Alprazolam, Xanax®, Pfizer Inc.

Amifostine, Ethyol®, Medimmune Oncology

Aminocaproic acid, Amicar®, Xanodyne Pharmaceuticals

Amitriptyline, Elavil®, AstraZeneca

Amoxicillin, Amoxil®, GlaxoSmithKline

Atenolol, Tenormin®, AstraZeneca

Atomoxetine, Strattera®, Eli Lilly and Co.

Azithromycin, Zithromax®, Pfizer Inc.

Baclofen, Lioresal®, Medtronic, Inc.

Beclomethasone, QVAR®, Teva Specialty Pharmaceuticals

Benzonatate, Tessalon Perles®, Forest Laboratories

Bisacodyl suppository, Dulcolax®, Boehringer Ingelheim

Bupropion sustained-release, Wellbutrin® SR, GlaxoSmithKline

Buspirone, BuSpar®, Bristol-Myers Squibb

Budesonide, Pulmicort Respules®, AstraZeneca

Carbamazepine, Tegretol®, Novartis

Casanthrol and docusate sodium, Peri-Colace®, Purdue Pharma L.P.

Cefotaxime, Claforan®, Sanofi-Aventis

Cefuroxime, Ceftin®, GlaxoSmithKline

Cephalexin, Keflex®, Middlebrook Pharmaceuticals

Cetirizine, Zyrtec®, Pfizer Inc.

Cevimeline, Evoxac®, Daiichi Sankyo, Inc.

Chlordiazepoxide, Librax®, Librium®, Limbitrol®, Valeant Pharmaceuticals

Chlorpromazine, Thorazine®, GlaxoSmithKline

Cholestyramine, Questran®, Bristol-Myers Squibb

Cimetidine, Tagamet®, GlaxoSmithKline

Ciprofloxacin, Cipro®, Bayer Pharmaceuticals

Citalopram, Celexa®, Forest Laboratoriess

Clomipramine, Anafranil®, Tyco Healthcare

Clonazepam, Klonopin®, Roche Pharmaceuticals

Clopidogrel, Plavix®, Sanofi-Aventis

Clorazepate, Tranxene®, Ovation Pharmaceuticals

Clozapine, Clozaril®, Novartis Collagenase; Santyl®, Advance Biofactures

Crotamiton, Eurax®, Ranbaxy Laboratories

Cyproheptadine, multiple manufacturers

Darbepoetin alfa, Aranesp®, Amgen Inc.

Demeclocycline, Declomycin®, Stiefel

Dexamethasone, multiple manufacturers

Dexmethylphenidate, Focalin®, Novartis

Dextroamphetamine, Dexedrine®, Smith-Kline Beecham; Adderall®, Shire US Inc.

Diazepam, Valium®, Roche Pharmaceuticals

Diphenhydramine, Benadryl®, McNeil

Diphenoxylate, Lomotil®, Pfizer Inc.

Dipyridamole, Persantine®, Boehringer Ingelheim

Disopyramide, Norpace®, GD Searle

Docusate, Colace®, Purdue Pharma L.P.

Donepezil, Aricept®, Eisai, Inc.

Doxazosin mesylate, Cardura®, Pfizer Inc.

Doxepin, Sinequan®, Pfizer Inc.

Doxycycline, Vibramycin®, Pfizer Inc.

Duloxetine, Cymbalta®, Eli Lilly and Co.

Epoetin alfa, Epogen®, Amgen Inc.; Procrit®, Ortho Biotech

Erythromycin, E-mycin®, Abbott Laboratories

Escitalopram, Lexapro®, Forest Laboratories

Estradiol, Estrace®, Bristol-Myers Squibb; Vagifem®, Novo Nordisk

Eszopiclone, Lunesta®, Sepracor

Famciclovir, Famvir®, Novartis

Famotidine, Pepcid®, Merck

Filgrastim, Neupogen®, Amgen Inc.

Flavoxate, Urispas®, Ortho-McNeil

Fluconazole, Diflucan®, Pfizer Inc.

Flunisolide, AeroBid®, Forest Laboratories

Fluoxetine, Prozac®, Eli Lilly and Co.

Fluticasone, Flovent®, GlaxoSmithKline

Fluvoxamine, Luvox®, Solvay Pharmaceuticals

Formoterol, Foradil®, Novartis

Furosemide, Lasix®, Sanofi-Aventis

Gabapentin, Neurontin®, Pfizer Inc.

Glutamine, L-glutamine, multiple manufacturers

Glycopyrrolate, Robinul®, Baxter Healthcare

Haloperidol, Haldol®, Johnson & Johnson

Hyaluronidase, Wydase®, Baxter Healthcare

Hydroxyzine, Vistaril®, Pfizer Inc.

Hyoscyamine, Levsin®, Alaven Pharmaceutical

Imipramine, Tofranil®, Tyco Healthcare

Ipratropium, Atrovent®, Boehringer Ingelheim

Ipratropium/albuterol, DuoNeb®, Dey, L.P.

Isoproterenol, Isuprel®, Hospira

Lactulose, Chronulac®, Sanofi-Aventis

Lansoprazole, Prevacid®, Tap Pharmaceutical Products, Inc.

Levofloxacin, Levaquin®, Ortho-McNeil

Lidocaine, Lidoderm®, Teikoku Pharma. USA

Loperamide, Imodium®, McNeil Consumer Healthcare

Loratadine, Claritin®, Schering-Plough

Lorazepam, Ativan®, Biovail

Methyldopa, Aldomet®, Merck

Methylphenidate, Ritalin®, Novartis

Methyltestosterone, Android®, Valeant Pharmacueticals Inc.

Methylprednisolone, Medrol®, Pfizer Inc.

Metoclopramide, Reglan®, Tablet: Schwarz Pharma; Injection: Baxter Healthcare

Metoproterenol, Alupent®, Boehringer Ingelheim

Metronidazole, Metrogel®, Galderma Laboratories

Midazolam, multiple manufacturers

Mirtazapine, Remeron®, Organon USA, Inc.

Modafinil, Provigil®, Cephalon

Mometasone, Asmanex®, Schering Corporation

Montelukast, Singulair®, Merck

Naloxone, multiple manufacturers

Nefazodone, multiple manufacturers

Nitrofurantoin, Macrodantin®, Procter & Gamble

Nortriptyline, Pamelor®, Tyco Healthcare

Nystatin, Mycostatin®, Ranbaxy Apothecon

Octreotide, Sandostatin®, Novartis

Ofloxacin, Floxin®, Ortho-McNeil

Olanzapine, Zyprexa®, Eli Lilly and Co.

Omeprazole, Prilosec®, AstraZeneca

Ondansetron, Zofran®, GlaxoSmithKline
Oxcarbazepine, Trileptal®, Novartis
Oxybutynin, Ditropan XL®, Alza Pharmaceuticals
Papain-urea, Accuzyme®, Healthpoint, Ltd.
Papain-urea-chlorophyllin copper complex sodium, Panafil®, Healthpoint, Ltd.
Paroxetine, Paxil®, GlaxoSmithKline
Phenazopyridine, Pyridium®, Mylan Labs
Phenytoin, Dilantin®, Mylan Labs
Pilocarpine, Salagen®, MGI Pharmaceuticals
Polycarbophil, Replens®, Lil' Drug Store Products, Inc.
Polyethylene glycol, Miralax®, Schering-Plough
Prednisone, Deltasone®, Pfizer Inc.
Propiverine, Detrunorm®, Amdipharm
Propranolol, Inderal®, Wyeth Pharmaceuticals, Inc.
Psyllium fiber supplement, Metamucil®, Procter & Gamble
Ranitidine, Zantac®, GlaxoSmithKline
Rifampin, Rifadin®, Sanofi-Aventis
Risperidone, Risperdal®, Janssen Pharma
Saline enema, Fleet®, C.B. Fleet Co. Inc.
Salmeterol, Serevent®, GlaxoSmithKline
Sargramostim, Leukine®, Bayer Healthcare Pharmaceuticals
Scopolamine, Transderm-Scop®, Novartis
Senna, Senokot®, Purdue Pharma L.P.
Senna concentrate and docusate sodium, Senokot® S, Purdue Pharma L.P.
Sertraline, Zoloft®, Pfizer Inc.
Sildenafil, Viagra®, Pfizer Inc.
Spironolactone, Aldactone®, Pfizer Inc.
Sulfamethoxazole, Bactrim®, Mutual Pharmaceutical Co.
Tacrine, Cognex®, Sciele Pharma, Inc.
Tamsulosin, Flomax®, Boehringer Ingelheim
Temazepam, Restoril®, Tyco Healthcare
Terazosin hydrochloride, Hytrin®, Abbott Laboratories
Terbinafine, Lamisil®, Novartis
Theophylline, Theo-Dur®, Schering-Plough
Thiothixene, Navane®, Pfizer Inc.
Ticlopidine, Ticlid®, Roche Pharmaceuticals

Tiotropium, Spiriva®, Boehringer Ingelheim
Tolterodine, Detrol® LA, Pfizer Inc.
Triamcinolone, Azmacort®, Abbott Laboratories
Triazolam, Halcion®, Pfizer Inc.
Trospium, Sanctura®, Indevus
Valacyclovir, Valtrex®, GlaxoSmithKline
Valproic acid, Depakene®, Abbott Laboratories
Vardenafil, Levitra®, Bayer Pharmaceuticals
Venlafaxine, Effexor®, Wyeth Pharmaceuticals, Inc.
Zafirlukast, Accolate®, AstraZeneca
Zaleplon, Sonata®, King Pharmaceuticals
Zolpidem tartrate, Ambien®, Sanofi-Aventis

Additional Brand-Name Products Mentioned and Their Manufacturers
Aveeno®, Johnson & Johnson
Bag Balm®, Dairy Association Company, Inc.
Balmex®, Chattem, Inc.
Banish®, Smith & Nephew
Biotene® Oral Balance®, Laclede
CarboFlex® Odor-Control Dressing, ConvaTec
Dove®, Unilever
Eucerin®, Beiersdorf, Inc.
Exuderm® OdorShield™, Medline Industries, Inc.
Gatorade®, PepsiCo
Gelfoam®, Galderma Laboratories
Hex-On®, Coloplast
Lubriderm®, McNeill-PPC, Ltd.
Maalox-Plus®, Novartis Consumer Health
Moi-Stir®, Kingwood Labs
Pedialyte®, Abbott Laboratories
Prosure®, Ross Products Division, Abbott Laboratories
QR Powder®, Biolife
Resource Support®, Novartis Medical Nutrition, Novartis Pharmaceuticals
Salivart®, Xenex Laboratories
Sarna®, Stiefel Canada, Inc.
Surgicel®, Johnson & Johnson
Zassi®, Zassi Medical Evolutions

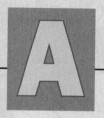

Advance Directives

Anemia

Anorexia, Cachexia, and
Nutrition Support

Anxiety

Ascites

Advance Directives

Crystal Dea Moore, PhD, MSW, MA

Definitions

Advance directives allow for the expression of end-of-life care medical wishes in the event that patients are unable to communicate these preferences as a result of incapacity. Advance directives, a form of extended autonomy, can take on three forms: oral directives, a written instructional directive, and a durable power of attorney for health care (also referred to as a healthcare proxy in some states) (Lo, 2004). *Living wills* are specific written instructions about the kinds of health care that should be provided or forgone in particular healthcare situations. A *durable power of attorney for health care* or *healthcare proxy* is a document that appoints an agent the person trusts to make decisions in the event of the appointing person's subsequent decisional incapacity. In some states, oral advance directives do not meet the criteria of "clear and convincing evidence" needed to legally document patient treatment preferences. Advance directives are part of the ongoing advance care planning process whereby patients, family members, decision-making surrogates, and healthcare professionals collaboratively clarify patient goals, values, and preferences about future healthcare treatments.

Specific Issues Related to Palliative Care

Conversations related to advance care planning can be difficult for a myriad of complicated reasons. Medical culture has been characterized as "valu[ing] technology over discussion" (Lynn et al., 2000, p. 218), and some medical professionals may be concerned that frank and open discussion about end-of-life care issues can diminish patient and family hope (Steinhauser et al., 2001). Waiting for the clinician to take the lead, patients may be reluctant to bring up advance care planning issues themselves, although researchers indicate that most patients want to be fully informed about their condition and prognosis (Jenkins, Fallowfield, & Saul, 2001; Steinhauser et al.).

The author would like to acknowledge Carol Taylor, CSFN, RN, PhD, for her contributions that remain unchanged from the first edition of this textbook.

Without timely, meaningful, and ongoing advance care planning, families relate narratives of their loved ones' dying being needlessly prolonged by undesired treatment or being hastened when treatment is withheld or withdrawn. Patients realistically fear that they will lose control of decision making as their voices can be stifled or ignored when they want aggressive therapy to be withheld or discontinued or when they demand aggressive life-sustaining therapy that a clinician judges to be medically futile. Factors contributing to physician reluctance to withhold or withdraw life-sustaining therapy include lack of familiarity with ethical and legal guidelines for withholding and withdrawing medical treatment, misunderstandings about the legal consequences of withholding or withdrawing treatment, failure to embrace preparation for a comfortable and dignified death as a legitimate aim of medicine, and a general lack of ease in initiating discussions about the plan of care as a patient's condition declines. Advances in knowledge and technology have proliferated treatment options and complicated healthcare decision making for many conditions. Patients and families need ongoing and easily understood education about treatment options so that they can make informed decisions about the direction of treatment.

In the context of modern healthcare systems, numerous obstacles to engaging in advance care planning exist, but the benefits of purposefully including these discussions over the course of treatment outweigh the costs. As part of this collaborative process, advance directive documents can be drafted and the medical team educated about the patient's end-of-life care wishes as the illness trajectory progresses, not just during the final throes of the illness. The completion of advance directives is not a one-time event. As patient preferences can and do change, particularly when a substantial change occurs in the patient's condition and/or quality of life, the documents should be revisited and revised as needed. Clinicians should educate themselves about patient and family cultural values and backgrounds as they relate to and influence end-of-life care issues and the actual completion of advance directives. For example, some cultural groups may prefer not to have direct discussions about diagnosis and prognosis, particularly if the outlook is grim (Van Winkle, 2000; Yeo & Hikoyeda, 2000).

Support for and Barriers to Advance Care Planning

A. Support for advance care planning (Emanuel, von Gunten, & Ferris, 1999): Common law, federal and state legislation, and official policies of medical organizations support advance care planning.
   1. U.S. Supreme Court, 1990 (in the case of Nancy Cruzan): The court upheld the patient's right to self-determination, establishing that the right applies even to patients who are no longer able to direct their own health care and that decisions for incompetent patients should be based on their previously stated wishes.
   2. Federal law, 1990: The Patient Self-Determination Act (PSDA) requires that patients be informed of their rights to accept or refuse medical treatment and to specify, in advance, the care they would like to receive should they become incapacitated.

3. State law: The patient's right to specify wishes in advance has been codified into statute in all 50 states, but state policies vary widely. Statutory documents recognized by law include the living will and the durable power of attorney for health care (i.e., healthcare proxy). Some states also have policy that gives family members, stated in an explicit hierarchy, the right to make decisions for a decisionally incapacitated patient in the absence of written documents.

4. Statutory documents: These documents are specifically described and defined in state statutes to help to protect clinicians who honor a patient's wishes. When such documents are used, rights, obligations, and protections are clearly defined.

5. Nonstatutory or advisory documents: These are legal and based on common law rights. They are intended to accurately reflect a patient's wishes. In some states or settings, an advisory document is enough; in others, a statutory form should be used, as well. In some states, a legal guardian may be necessary if no statutory power of attorney exists for health care.

6. Professional policy
   a) In 1997, the American Medical Association's Council on Ethical and Judicial Affairs identified advance care planning as an essential component of standard medical practice. It called for physicians to conduct advance planning discussions on a routine basis, using advisory documents as an adjunct to statutory documents, such as the living will and the durable power of attorney for health care. The American College of Physicians' (2005) *Ethics Manual* also supports advance care planning.
   b) The American Nurses Association (ANA) has a position statement on nursing and the PSDA. The ANA (1991) position is that "nurses should play a primary role in implementation of the PSDA. It is the responsibility of nurses to facilitate informed decision making for patients making choices about end-of-life care. The clinician's role in education, research, patient care, and advocacy is critical to implementation of the PSDA within all healthcare settings."

B. Explanations for the failure of many to execute advance directives
   1. Drafting an advance directive means admitting one's mortality; this is an uncomfortable subject for many in our death-denying culture.
   2. Healthcare professionals may wait for patients to initiate conversation about advance directives, and patients also may wait for healthcare professionals to do the same.
   3. Advance care planning takes time. Given clinical time constraints and the fragmented nature of the modern healthcare system, healthcare professionals may see themselves as "too busy" to have these conversations, and advance care planning does not have an *International Classification of Diseases* code.
   4. Some people may fear that the mere existence of an advance directive will prejudice healthcare professionals to withhold desired care.

Strategies to Promote Use of Advance Directives in Palliative Care

A. Familiarize yourself with state and institutional policies that address the completion and implementation of advance directives.

B. Educate the public and healthcare professionals about advance directives.

C. Incorporate advance care planning discussions into everyday patient care, including family members and decision-making surrogates whenever possible. Address not only issues related to specific medical treatments but also patient goals and values, which can inform the medical care plan. See Figure 1-1 for suggested questions to promote advance care planning discussions.

D. Make advance directives a part of the medical record, and ensure that all parties (i.e., the patient, the decision-making surrogate, family members) understand the implications for treatment and care (American Hospital Association, 1991).

E. Presume nothing about an advance directive until you have read it carefully. For patients with completed advance directives, review and discuss the contents with the patient and, if applicable, the designated surrogate and/or family members.

F. Resolve implementation problems, including
   1. Conflicts about when an advance directive becomes operative
   2. Conflicts when an attending clinician elects to ignore advance directives
   3. Conflicts when designated surrogates ignore patient preferences documented in an advance directive
   4. Conflicts about how to interpret the content of the directive.

Patient Outcomes

A. A documented record exists of the patient's preferences for end-of-life care and identification and contact information of the person the patient trusts to make his or her decisions should the patient lack decisional capacity.

B. Advance care planning discussions can promote shared decision making and a stronger sense of patient control over the dying process.

C. Clearly developed advance directives and inclusive advance care planning discussions can decrease conflict over the directions of the patient's future care.

Evaluating the Evidence

A. Conflicting evidence exists about the number of adults who have completed advance directives. Estimates range from less than 25% (Emanuel, Barry,

Figure 1-1. Suggested Questions for Advance Care Planning Discussions

Patient Understanding of Illness
- What do you understand about the current state of your illness? (Lo et al., 1999)
- What do you know about your treatment options?

Patient Preferences Regarding Information Delivery
- How much do you want to know about your illness?
- Who would you like to be present during such discussions?

Considerations in Choosing Decision-Making Surrogates
- Who would you want to make decisions for you if something happened and you were unable to make decisions about your care?
- Have you spoken with this person about being your decision maker? Have you discussed your wishes with him or her?
- Have you informed other important people in your life about your choice of decision maker?
- How well do you think this person can deal with any disagreements others may have about your wishes?
- If you anticipate any disagreements, what do you believe the best way is to address this?
- To what extent do you want your family and loved ones to have input in decisions that are made about your health care?
- How important is it that your family as a whole agrees with the decisions that are made on your behalf?

Patient Goals
- What is important for you to accomplish at this point in your life?
- As you think about the future, what is most important to you (what matters the most to you)? (Lo et al., 1999)
- What are your hopes and fears for the future?
- If you were to die sooner rather than later, what would be left undone? (Quill, 2000)
- What type of legacy do you want to leave your family and loved ones? (Lo et al., 1999)

Patient Values
- What makes life worth living? (Quill, 2000)
- What would have to happen for your life to be not worth living?
- What nourishes your spirit?
- How do you feel about quality versus quantity of life?
- What are your thoughts about pain control? Would you want your pain controlled even if it meant that you might not be as alert?

Personal Experiences With Illness, Death, and Dying
- Has anyone close to you died of an illness? What happened? What was it like for you?
- What other significant losses have you experienced?
- What would you consider a "good death"?

Spirituality and Existential Issues
- What thoughts have you had about why you got this illness at this time? (Lo et al., 1999)
- Is faith (religion, spirituality) important to you in this illness, and has it been important to you at other times in your life? (Lo et al., 1999)
- Would you like to explore religious or spiritual matters with someone? Do you have someone to talk to about these things? (Lo et al., 1999)
- Do you have any spiritual or religious beliefs that should be taken into consideration by your healthcare providers?

Note. From "Communication Issues and Advance Care Planning," by C.D. Moore, 2005, *Seminars in Oncology Nursing, 21,* p. 18. Copyright 2005 by Elsevier. Adapted with permission.

Stoeckle, Ettelson, & Emanuel, 1991; Hanson & Rodgman, 1996; Lo, 2004) to 71% (Teno, Gruneir, Schwartz, Nanda, & Wetle, 2007).

B. Evidence from the seminal SUPPORT study (Study to Understand Prognoses and Preferences for Outcomes and Risks of Treatment) indicate that advance directives have a limited role in guiding patient care (SUPPORT Principal Investigators, 1995).

C. Consistent with other more recent findings, one national study found that written advance directives were associated with "less use of life-sustaining treatment, greater use of hospice, and less likelihood of terminal hospitalization" (Teno et al., 2007, p. 192).

Resources

Advance directives and supporting information may be obtained from the following sources.

A. American Academy of Family Physicians: http://familydoctor.org

B. National Hospice and Palliative Care Organization: www.caringinfo.org

C. Aging With Dignity and Five Wishes: www.agingwithdignity.org

References

American College of Physicians. (2005). *Ethics manual* (5th ed.). Philadelphia: Author.

American Hospital Association. (1991). *Put it in writing: A guide to promoting advance directives*. Chicago: Author.

American Nurses Association. (1991). *Ethics and human rights position statements: Nursing and the Patient Self-Determination Act*. Retrieved May 1, 2007, from http://nursingworld.org/readroom/position/ethics/etsdet.htm

Emanuel, L.L., Barry, M.J., Stoeckle, J.D., Ettelson, L.M., & Emanuel, E. (1991). Advance directives for medical care—A case of greater use. *New England Journal of Medicine, 324,* 889–895.

Emanuel, L.L., von Gunten, C.F., & Ferris, F.D. (1999). *The education for physicians on end-of-life care (EPEC) curriculum*. Princeton, NJ: The Robert Wood Johnson Foundation.

Hanson, L.C., & Rodgman, E. (1996). The use of living wills at the end of life: A national study. *Archives of Internal Medicine, 156,* 1018–1022.

Jenkins, V.A., Fallowfield, L.J., & Saul, J. (2001). Information needs of patients with cancer: Results from a large study in UK cancer centres. *British Journal of Cancer, 84,* 48–51.

Lo, B. (2004). Advance care planning. *American Journal of Geriatric Cardiology, 19,* 316–320.

Lo, B., Quill, T.E., & Tulsky, J.A. (1999). Discussing palliative care with patients. *Annals of Internal Medicine, 130,* 744–749.

Lynn, J., Arkes, H.R., Stevens, M., Cohn, F., Koenig, B., Fox, E., et al. (2000). Rethinking fundamental assumptions: SUPPORTS's implications for future reform. *Journal of the American Geriatrics Society, 48,* 214–221.

Patient Self-Determination Act of 1990, H.R. 5835 [OBRA 1990], 101st Congress (1990).

Quill, T.E. (2000). Initiating end-of-life discussions with seriously ill patients: Addressing the "elephant in the room." *JAMA, 284,* 2502–2507.

Steinhauser, K.E., Christakis, N.A., Clipp, E.C., McNeilly, M., Grambow, S., Parker, J., et al. (2001). Preparing for the end of life: Preferences of patients, families, physicians, and other care providers. *Journal of Pain and Symptom Management, 22,* 727–737.

SUPPORT Principal Investigators. (1995). A controlled trial to improve care for seriously ill hospitalized patients: The study to understand prognoses and preferences of outcomes and risks of treatments. *JAMA, 274,* 1591–1598.

Teno, J.M., Gruneir, A., Schwartz, Z., Nanda, A., & Wetle, T. (2007). Association between advance directives and quality of end-of-life care: A national study. *Journal of the American Geriatrics Society, 55,* 189–194.

Van Winkle, N.W. (2000). End-of-life decision making in American Indian and Alaska Native cultures. In K. Braun, J. Pietsch, & P. Blanchette (Eds.), *Cultural issues in end-of-life decision making* (pp. 127–144). Thousand Oaks, CA: Sage.

Yeo, G., & Hikoyeda, N. (2000). Cultural issues in end-of-life decision making among Asians and Pacific Islanders in the United States. In K. Braun, J. Pietsch, & P. Blanchette (Eds.), *Cultural issues in end-of-life decision making* (pp. 101–126). Thousand Oaks, CA: Sage.

Anemia

Joyce Marrs, MS, FNP-BC, AOCNP®

Definition

Anemia is a decrease in the number of circulating red blood cells resulting from some underlying disorder. It may be seen as an acute or chronic condition.

Pathophysiology and Etiology

Patients with cancer or chronic illness often develop anemia. The cause is generally multifactorial and may include chemotherapy treatment, radiation therapy, nutritional deficits, blood loss, or damaged bone marrow (Dunn, Carter, & Carter, 2003; Griffin, 2001). Although no data exist to support a direct correlation between fatigue scores and hemoglobin level, the resulting overall effect of anemia can severely affect the patient's quality of life (Munch, Zhang, Willey, Palmer, & Bruera, 2005). Appropriate treatment of anemia as part of palliative care should be based on the uniqueness of each patient's situation.

Manifestations

- Fatigue
- Weakness
- Shortness of breath: pulmonary edema and congestive heart failure possible
- Malaise
- Dizziness/orthostasis
- Headache
- Cold intolerance
- Tachycardia/tachypnea
- Palpitations
- Pallor
- Depression

The author would like to acknowledge Peg Esper, MSN, MSA, RN, AOCN®, APRN-BC, for her contribution that remains unchanged from the first edition of this textbook.

- Cognitive changes
(Davis, 2004; Loney & Chernecky, 2000)

Management

The goal of treatment is to correct anemia. An increase in hemoglobin level will promote improved quality of life through enhanced physical, emotional, and cognitive function (Dunn et al., 2003). Extent of testing and treatment is based upon survival expectancy and disease status (Davis, 2004).

A. Death is not imminent.
  1. **Level I—high level of evidence**
     a) Oral iron supplements ($)—Ferrous sulfate, 325 mg po tid. Beneficial if the individual is iron deficient. Iron deficiency is typically identified through a low serum ferritin level. However, a serum ferritin level can be raised by conditions such as inflammation, malignancy, and liver disease, which may mask iron deficiency. Although readily available and inexpensive to administer, iron supplements can have a number of unpleasant side effects, such as gastrointestinal upset and constipation. Should a patient have difficulty with oral iron, administration of IV iron is an option (Davis, 2004).
     b) Blood transfusion ($$)—Administration early in care often can palliate symptoms but also may provide no benefit. Patient evaluation post-transfusion should occur to evaluate for a decrease in symptoms. In situations where bone marrow is compromised, blood transfusions serve a very temporary benefit, if any. Careful justification of transfusion should be made before initiating this treatment (Monti, Castellani, Berlusconi, & Cunietti, 1996).
     c) Erythropoietin administration ($$$)—Use of erythropoietin agents is debatable in palliative care settings. Their use may decrease cancer-related fatigue but may not benefit all individuals. Weekly injections include side effects such as fever, chills, and bone pain. The benefit generally is not seen for several weeks following initiation of treatment and requires that patients have adequate ferritin levels for it to be effective (Micromedex, 2001). Concurrent administration of iron is recommended. Hematocrit levels should be checked regularly, twice a week for two to six weeks following any dose adjustment. Dose reduction should be made if hemoglobin increase is more than 1 g/dl in a two-week period. Because of the risk of severe and life-threatening cardiovascular events, target hemoglobin level should be within a range of 10–12 g/dl (U.S. Food and Drug Administration Alert, 2006). Anemia that fails to respond to erythropoietin agents is indicative of a poor prognosis (Davis, 2004). The cost of this agent may not be covered by the patient's insurance. Anticipated benefits should be evaluated carefully prior to use in this setting. When a target

hemoglobin of ≥ 12 g/dl is maintained, clinical trials demonstrated that overall survival and/or time to tumor progression may be decreased (U.S. Food and Drug Administration Alert, 2007).

2. **Level II—moderate level of evidence**

   Folic acid ($)—Folic acid 1,000 mcg po daily. A portion of patients with anemia in the palliative care setting have folic acid deficiency (Dunn et al., 2003). The body stores of folic acid can be depleted within four to five months. Although little research supporting this intervention exists, the prevalence was identified through a prospective audit involving 105 patients, and administration of folic acid should be considered for patients with a documented deficiency (Dunn et al.).

B. Death is imminent.

   Level III—low level of evidence
   1. Attempts to treat manifestations of the anemia and not the anemia itself should be instituted.
   2. Interventions include oxygen (use a nasal cannula, as masks often make people feel as though they are suffocating), rest, warm clothing, and blankets. Avoid sudden movements.

Patient Outcomes

A. Anemia is corrected when feasible.

B. Anemia-associated symptoms are relieved.

C. Quality of life is improved.

References

Davis, M. (2004). Hematology in palliative medicine. *American Journal of Hospice and Palliative Medicine, 21,* 445–454.

Dunn, A., Carter, J., & Carter, H. (2003). Anemia at the end of life: Prevalence, significance, and causes in patients receiving palliative care. *Journal of Pain and Symptom Management, 26,* 1132–1139.

Griffin, J.D. (2001). Hematopoietic growth factors. In V.T. DeVita, S. Hellman, & S.A. Rosenberg (Eds.), *Cancer: Principles and practice of oncology* (6th ed., pp. 2798–2813). Philadelphia: Lippincott Williams & Wilkins.

Loney, M., & Chernecky, C. (2000). Anemia. *Oncology Nursing Forum, 27,* 951–962.

Micromedex. (2001). *Healthcare series.* Greenwood Village, CO: Author.

Monti, M., Castellani, L., Berlusconi, A., & Cunietti, E. (1996). Use of red blood cell transfusion in terminally ill cancer patients admitted to a palliative care unit. *Journal of Pain and Symptom Management, 12,* 18–22.

Munch, T., Zhang, T., Willey, J., Palmer, J., & Bruera, E. (2005). The association between anemia and fatigue in patients with advanced cancer receiving palliative care. *Journal of Palliative Medicine, 8,* 1144–1149.

U.S. Food and Drug Administration Alert. (2006, November 16). *Information for healthcare professionals: Erythropoiesis stimulating agents (ESA).* Retrieved April 15, 2007, from http://www.fda.gov/cder/drug/InfoSheets/HCP/RHE2007HCP.htm

U.S. Food and Drug Administration Alert. (2007, November 8). *Information on erythropoiesis agents (ESA)*. Retrieved November 27, 2007, from http://www.fda.gov/cder/drug/infopage/RHE/default.htm

Anorexia, Cachexia, and Nutrition Support

Suzanne Dixon, MPH, MS, RD, and
Peg Esper, MSN, MSA, RN, AOCN®, APRN-BC

Definitions

Anorexia is a lack of appetite resulting in an involuntary decline of food intake. *Cachexia,* of which anorexia is typically a feature, encompasses the disordered metabolism characteristic of certain diseases or conditions. Common causes of cachexia include cancer, sepsis, chronic infections, HIV/AIDS, liver disease, and other conditions resulting in systemic inflammation. Cachexia and subsequent anorexia can lead to weight loss, loss of lean body mass and functional status, and decline in quality of life for patients with advanced illness. Cachexia is reported as the main cause of death in 20% of patients with advanced cancer (Del Fabbro, Dalal, & Bruera, 2006).

Pathophysiology and Etiology

Patients with advanced cancer often develop cachexia and subsequent anorexia. The cause of cachexia is not completely understood; recent data suggest that derangements in the lysosomal system, the ubiquitin-proteasome pathway, and cytosolic proteases may contribute to its development (Melstrom, Melstrom, Ding, & Adrian, 2007). Of these three mechanisms, the ubiquitin-proteasome pathway may account for the majority of skeletal muscle degradation in cancer cachexia through the action of cytokines, including tumor necrosis factor-alpha, interleukin-1 beta, interleukin-6, interferon-gamma, and proteolysis-inducing factor (Bhogal, Lorite, & Tisdale, 2006; Kuroda et al., 2007; Melstrom et al.; Skipworth, Stewart, Dejong, Preston, & Fearon, 2007). Additionally, new research points to alterations in the dystrophin glycoprotein complex as an important early event in the development of cachexia (Acharyya & Guttridge, 2007).

Regardless of the cause, it is clear that cachexia contributes to anorexia, hypermetabolism, and alterations in normal metabolic pathways. In simple starvation, the body readily adapts to calorie deficit by shifting to fatty acids as a major source of energy, thereby preserving lean body mass. In the cachectic state, the body fails to make this adaptation, which can lead to disproportionate wasting of lean body mass and loss of strength and functional status. This results in a marked decline in quality of life for individuals with terminal illness (Fornari & McCallum, 2006; Hutton et al., 2006; MacDonald, 2007; Marin Caro, Laviano, & Pichard, 2007; Melstrom et al., 2007). An understanding of this process is important because even in patients who are overweight or obese, cachexia-related weight loss will decrease lean body mass and quality of life and should be addressed in order to provide optimal palliative care.

Manifestations

- Anorexia
- Weight loss
- Lean body mass loss
- Weakness
- Early satiety
- Malaise
- Anemia
- Dehydration
- Electrolyte imbalances
- Taste alterations
- Xerostomia
- Nausea
- Fatigue
- Lethargy
- Micronutrient deficiency
- Thyroid dysfunction

Management

A. Death is not imminent.
　　1. **Level I—high level of evidence**
　　　　a) Megestrol acetate ($$)—Megestrol acetate is a synthetic progestational agent with a long history of use for treating anorexia and weight loss associated with cancer cachexia. Several clinical trials have been conducted on the use of megestrol acetate to manage anorexia and weight loss in a variety of populations, but most predominantly in patients with cancer cachexia. Two comprehensive reviews, a Cochrane Database review, and a meta-analysis concluded that this medication is effective and beneficial for managing anorexia associated with cachexia in advanced cancer cases (Berenstein & Ortiz, 2005; Mateen & Jatoi, 2006; Melstrom et al., 2007; Pascual et al., 2004). Typical dosing for megestrol acetate is 800 mg (20 ml oral suspension) po once daily, taken in the morning (Von Roenn, 2006).
　　　　b) Referral to a registered dietitian ($)—Referral to a registered dietitian can improve nutritional status and outcomes for patients who are treated palliatively or with curative intent. Several controlled trials demonstrated

that for better symptom management and improved outcomes in oncology populations, dietitian-delivered nutrition intervention was superior to usual nutrition care by other healthcare professionals. Individuals randomized to receive intensive nutrition intervention, dietitian-guided nutritional management, or the American Dietetic Association Medical Nutrition Therapy protocol lost significantly less weight; had significantly smaller deteriorations in global quality of life, physical functioning, and nutrition status; and were significantly more satisfied with the quality of overall cancer and nutrition care as compared to patients randomized to receive usual (non-dietitian-directed) nutrition care (Isenring, Bauer, & Capra, 2007; Isenring, Capra, & Bauer, 2004a, 2004b; Odelli et al., 2005; Ravasco, Monteiro-Grillo, Marques Vidal, & Camilo, 2005). In curative oncology care, nutrition intervention contributes to reduced postoperative infection rates, better cancer-related symptom control, decreased length of hospital stays, and improved treatment tolerance. In palliative care, nutrition intervention focuses on controlling symptoms and improving quality of life (Marin Caro, Laviano, & Pichard, 2007).

2. **Level II—moderate level of evidence**
   a) Insulin ($$)—One controlled clinical trial in a palliative care setting demonstrated that insulin therapy can significantly increase dietary intake, decrease serum free fatty acids, improve metabolic efficiency during exertion, and improve quality of life without apparent stimulation of tumor growth. Data indicate an effective dose of 0.11 +/– 0.05 units/kg/day with blood glucose monitoring as required to further guide dosing (Lundholm et al., 2007).
   b) Oxandrolone ($$)—Two small controlled trials of oxandrolone, a synthetic oral anabolic agent, demonstrated that this medication increases weight and lean body mass, as well as quality of life and performance status in patients with cancer-related weight loss (Boughton, 2003; Von Roenn, Tchekmedyian, Sheng, & Ottery, 2002). Oxandrolone is contraindicated for use in patients with breast and prostate cancer who have hypercalcemia, or in any individual with severe hepatic dysfunction or nephrosis. It should be used with caution in conjunction with warfarin and in patients with existing cardiac, renal, or hepatic disease (Von Roenn, 2006). Typical dosing for oxandrolone is 10 mg po bid.
   c) Dronabinol ($$)—Dronabinol is a synthetic version of delta-9-THC (delta-9-tetrahydrocannabinol), a naturally occurring compound found in marijuana that is responsible for its orexigenic effects. Dronabinol is administered po and is approved for chemotherapy-induced nausea and vomiting in patients with cancer who have failed to respond adequately to conventional treatments and for treating patients with AIDS-related anorexia and weight loss (Solvay Pharmaceuticals, 2007). Data demonstrate that dronabinol is well tolerated (Cannabis-In-Cachexia-Study-Group et al., 2006) and possibly effective for treating anorexia associated with cancer- and AIDS-associated cachexia (Von Roenn, 2006; Walsh,

Nelson, & Mahmoud, 2003). Dronabinol should be used with caution in combination with other sedative and psychoactive medications. Typical dosing for dronabinol is 2.5 mg po two to three times per day. Initiating dronabinol at the lowest dose range and gradually increasing dosage will help to manage medication side effects and provide the best therapeutic outcomes (Von Roenn, 2006).

   d) Metoclopramide ($)—Use of metoclopramide, a prokinetic agent, may provide significant relief, lessen nausea and vomiting, lessen bloating, and improve appetite (Bruera et al., 2000; Wilson et al., 2002). One possible side effect of metoclopramide is diarrhea caused by hypermotility. A dose reduction or treatment with diphenhydramine will resolve this issue (Von Roenn, 2006). A suggested dosing schedule for metoclopramide is 10 mg four times per day (Von Roenn).

   e) Corticosteroids ($)—Decreased nausea, increased sense of well-being, and increased appetite have been documented, although no persistent increase in weight has been seen (Del Fabbro et al., 2006). The beneficial effects appear to be time limited and must be balanced against long-term side effects of administration, including Cushing syndrome, proximal myopathy, immunosuppression, and exacerbation of delirium.

3. **Level III—low level of evidence**

   a) Eicosapentaenoic acid (EPA), fish oil—Several phase I and phase II studies have demonstrated that EPA-enriched dietary supplements (Prosure®, Resource Support®) can ameliorate symptoms of cachexia, including weight loss and loss of lean body mass; other clinical trials have provided mixed results (Barber & Fearon, 2001; Barber, McMillan, Preston, Ross, & Fearon, 2000; Dewey, Baughan, Dean, Higgins, & Johnson, 2007; Fearon et al., 2003; Moses, Slater, Preston, Barber, & Fearon, 2004).

   b) General measures (patient tips)—Treat and manage symptoms affecting nutritional intake and desire to eat, including constipation; bloating; diarrhea; feelings of fullness, early satiety, and poor appetite; altered sense of taste or smell; dry mouth or thick saliva; sore mouth or throat; nausea or vomiting; and pain.

     (1) Constipation (See Constipation.)

     (2) Bloating

        (a) Limit beverages and foods that cause gas, such as carbonated drinks, broccoli, cabbage, cauliflower, cucumbers, peppers, beans, peas, onions, and garlic.

        (b) Lessen the amount of air swallowed by encouraging the patient to limit talking while eating.

        (c) Encourage the patient to avoid using straws to drink.

        (d) Encourage the patient to avoid chewing gum.

     (3) Diarrhea (See Diarrhea.)

     (4) Feelings of fullness, early satiety, and poor appetite

(a) Offer the patient several smaller meals and snacks each day instead of three larger meals.

(b) Make eating more enjoyable by setting an attractive table, playing favorite music, or watching television.

(c) Keep snacks handy for the patient to eat immediately (hunger may only last a few minutes), such as granola bars, nuts, pudding, chips, crackers, pretzels, trail mix, canned fruit, fresh fruit, and single-serving sizes of tuna or chicken.

(d) Offer favorite foods any time of the day (e.g., if breakfast foods are appealing to the patient, offer them for dinner).

(e) Encourage the patient to eat every few hours—do not wait for the patient to express feelings of hunger.

(f) Treat food like medicine—set times to eat, such as every one to two hours, and be sure the patient has at least a couple of bites of some food at each "medication" time. Quantity and type of food are less important; frequency of eating is more important.

(g) Offer high-calorie, high-protein drinks or fortified juice-based supplements.

(h) Offer fluids between meals rather than with meals (i.e., separate liquids from solids).

(i) Provide favorite foods and encourage the patient to be in control of food choices.

(j) Make dining area as appealing and pleasant as possible by removing bed pans, medication bottles, and the like.

(5) Altered sense of taste/smell

(a) Encourage the patient to be fastidious with mouth care.

(b) Avoid food smells.

(c) Avoid meal preparation by the patient.

(d) Try foods that have minimal odors and short cooking time, such as scrambled eggs, French toast, pancakes, oatmeal, and Cream of Wheat® (Nabisco).

(e) Season foods with tart flavors, such as lemon, citrus, and vinegar (avoid if sore mouth/throat is present).

(f) Flavor foods with basil, oregano, rosemary, tarragon, mustard, ketchup, or mint.

(g) Marinate and cook meats in sweet fruit juices, dressings, or wine, such as sweet and sour pork, chicken with honey glaze, or beef with burgundy wine or Italian dressing.

(h) Instruct the patient to rinse the mouth with tea, ginger ale, salted water, or baking soda and water to clear taste buds before eating.

(i) Offer the patient lemon drops, mints, or gum (avoid if sore mouth/throat is present; avoid sugarless gum and candy if diarrhea is present).

(6) Sore mouth and throat

(a) Encourage the patient to be fastidious with mouth care.

(b) Offer the patient bland foods, such as creamed soups, cooked cereals, macaroni and cheese, yogurt, pudding, mashed potatoes, eggs, custards, casseroles, cheesecake, and milk shakes.

(c) Instruct the patient to drink through a straw to bypass mouth sores.

(d) Offer high-protein, high-calorie foods to speed healing.

(e) Blend or moisten foods with olive oil, gravy, butter, cream, or sauces.

(f) Soften foods such as bread by soaking them in milk.

(g) Try nonacidic juices such as apple juice; peach, pear, or apricot nectars; and grape juice (do not use grape juice if diarrhea is present).

(h) Avoid offering the patient tart, acidic, or salty beverages and foods, such as citrus, pickled items, and tomato-based foods.

(i) Encourage the patient to avoid alcohol, caffeine, and tobacco.

(j) Avoid mouth care products that contain alcohol or other drying, irritating ingredients; try specialty mouth care products.

(7) Nausea and vomiting (See Nausea and Vomiting.)

(8) Dry mouth or thick saliva (See Xerostomia.)

(9) Pain (See Pain.)

4. **Level IV—inconclusive level of evidence**

   A number of randomized trials have been reported in the literature both supporting and refuting the use of artificial nutrition in palliative care (Hoda, Jatoi, Burnes, Loprinzi, & Kelly, 2005; Shang, Weiss, Post, & Kachler, 2006; Strasser & Bruera, 2002). As a result, the authors find the level of evidence for the use of artificial nutrition to be inconclusive at this time. Based on this, general guidelines concerning the use of various types of artificial nutrition will be presented.

   a) The American Dietetic Association recommends that the following issues be considered when deciding upon initiation or continuation of artificial nutrition support (Fornari & McCallum, 2006).

   (1) The patient's desire for nutrition intervention must be taken into account.

   (2) The decision to forgo hydration or nutrition support should be carefully contemplated because it may be difficult to reverse outcomes of following this path, even for a short period of time.

   (3) The benefits, risks, and burdens of nutrition support, including whether oral or parenteral nutrition will improve quality of life and well-being during the final stages of life, must be weighed.

   (4) Whether nutrition support will provide the patient with emotional comfort, decreased anxiety, relief from anorexia and cachexia, improved self-esteem, improved relationships with family and friends, and relief from fear of abandonment must be considered.

b) Enteral nutrition support ($$$) may be an option if
  (1) It can contribute to quality or length of life in a meaningful way.
  (2) The patient wants it.
  (3) The patient has a functioning gut.
  (4) It is not contraindicated by conditions such as intractable nausea and vomiting, obstruction, or gastroparesis (may be able to bypass these with a jejunal feeding tube instead of a gastric feeding tube).
c) Indications
  (1) The patient meets < 50% of required nutrient intake orally for five to seven days or more.
  (2) Inadequate oral intake occurs for five or more days.
  (3) Protein-energy malnutrition is present.
  (4) The patient is suffering from severe dysphagia.
d) Contraindications
  (1) The patient is diagnosed with an intestinal obstruction, ileus, or hypomotility of the intestine.
  (2) The patient has severe, intractable diarrhea that is unresponsive to treatment (i.e., treatment of underlying infection, diet modification, antidiarrheals).
  (3) High-output enterocutaneous fistula is present.
  (4) The patient is diagnosed with acute pancreatitis.
  (5) The prognosis does not warrant aggressive nutrition support; this is an individual decision that must be discussed with the patient and family and treated on a case-by-case basis.
e) Starting enteral feeding
  (1) A registered dietitian should be consulted to determine nutrient needs and to select a formula (e.g., high-protein, fiber-containing, elemental) and administration method (i.e., pump, gravity feeding, bolus feeding).
  (2) Micronutrient deficiencies should be addressed ($)—If death is not imminent, use of vitamin and mineral supplements, such as an iron supplement for iron-deficiency anemia (microcytic) or vitamin B_{12} and folic acid supplements for macrocytic/megaloblastic anemia, may be beneficial. However, the benefit of such supplementation must be weighed against the potential discomfort it can cause. It may be more beneficial to discontinue vitamin and mineral supplements that contribute to gastrointestinal distress, nausea, constipation, or diarrhea if they diminish quality of life by a significant degree (Fornari & McCallum, 2006). This issue must be discussed with the patient, family, and caregivers. The costs and benefits of micronutrient supplementation should be decided on a case-by-case basis.
d) Parenteral nutrition support ($$$$)—The most important issue is to help the family and patient to understand the risks, benefits, and cost of total parenteral nutrition on a case-by-case basis. Parenteral nutri-

tion is almost never indicated in the patient who is terminally ill for the following reasons.

(1) It adds very little in terms of quality and length of life.

(2) The risks (e.g., infection, hepatic and renal complications, fluid management problems) often outweigh the benefits.

(3) Treatment is very expensive.

(4) It requires frequent blood work (no less than weekly) and intensive management.

(5) It can contribute to other problems and complications, such as ascites, edema, and hepatic and renal complications.

B. Death is imminent.

1. Decreased food and fluid intake appears to be a normal part of the "physiology" of dying.

2. In the last few weeks to days of life, a marked decline occurs in the functioning of the upper and lower gastrointestinal system, as well as a decrease in sensations of taste and smell.

3. Education of family members and caregivers at this stage is important.

4. Facilitate understanding that the physical sensations of "starving" are not present. The patient feels little discomfort strictly from decreasing nutrition status. Hunger is nonexistent, and forcing the issue of food often is counterproductive.

5. Maintenance of strength and nutrition status at this time is unrealistic. Caregivers should be encouraged to show love and support in ways that do not involve preparation or provision of food.

6. Dehydration also may be normal during the end stage of the dying process. Often, the only discomfort associated with dehydration is a dry mouth, which can be alleviated with sips of water, ice chips, or moistened swabs (Fornari & McCallum, 2006). Explaining that dehydration is a normal part of the body shutting down in the final stages of life will ease the anxiety of caregivers. (See Dehydration.)

7. Artificial hydration and nutrition support at this time can decrease quality of life simply by the nature of their invasiveness. Starting these measures when death is imminent is not advised.

8. If artificial hydration or nutrition support is already in place, decreasing the amount of the infusion to 500–600 ml/day may help to avoid discomfort from increased urinary output, gastrointestinal and pharyngeal secretions, and pulmonary edema. Discontinuing hydration altogether is an option that should be determined by the patient and family (Fornari & McCallum, 2006).

9. According to the American Medical Association's Code of Ethics, human dignity is the primary obligation if it conflicts with prolonging life. All competent patients have the right to accept or reject any or all forms of medical treatment. If an advance directive is in place, this should specify the patient's desires with regard to supportive interventions, including fluids and artificial nutrition, at the end of life (American Medical Association, 2001).

10. If the patient expresses a desire for voluntary cessation of eating and drinking, the following issues must be considered and addressed (Byock, 2000; Miller, Fins, & Snyder, 2000; Quill & Byock, 2000a, 2000b).

   a) Patient characteristics: Persistent, unrelenting, otherwise-unrelieved symptoms that are deemed unacceptable to the patient and family, including pain, seizures, weakness, and extreme fatigue

   b) Patient informed consent
      (1) Patient must be fully competent.
      (2) Patient must be fully informed of all treatment and symptom management options.
      (3) Patient must be evaluated by a mental health professional to rule out treatable depression or other mental health conditions; a second opinion is strongly recommended.
      (4) A written informed consent must be in place.

   c) Terminal prognosis: Typically days to weeks (possibly months)

   d) Palliative care: Must be available, in place, and able to adequately relieve suffering

   e) Family participation: Clinicians should encourage discussion; consensus should be reached, if possible, among the patient, immediate family members, and caregivers.

   f) Patient incompetence: Food and fluids (oral) should not be denied from incompetent patients who are willing and able to eat.

   g) Second opinions: Must be obtained by experts in underlying disease, mental health, pain management, and palliative care.

11. If all of the aforementioned issues are addressed and managed, voluntary refusal of food and fluids may be an appropriate option. Artificial nutrition and hydration are considered life-sustaining medical therapies similar to medications, surgery, dialysis, mechanical ventilation, or other medical interventions. Therefore, decisions regarding this issue should be handled using the same ethical and legal standards as other interventions. If the benefits of an intervention outweigh the costs, it is justified. If it is not beneficial or if the costs are higher than the benefits, it is not justified. Discontinuation of nutrition and hydration generally is not considered justified in the following situations (Byock, 2000; Miller et al., 2000; National Comprehensive Cancer Network Nutrition Support Panel, 2006; Quill & Byock, 2000a, 2000b).

   a) The patient will die of malnutrition before he or she would succumb to the disease process. An example includes a patient with severe dysphagia secondary to head and neck cancer, in which the primary diagnosis will not result in death before malnutrition.

   b) Untreated mental health issues are present, such as depression.

   c) The patient has a strong desire to "get affairs in order," such as writing a will or attending a specific family event.

   d) A new acute, but treatable, diagnosis arises.

Patient Outcomes

A. Malnutrition, dehydration, micronutrient deficiencies, weakness, wasting, and weight loss are corrected when possible.

B. When maintenance of nutrition and hydration status is no longer a reasonable goal, comfort needs should be met.

C. Patient maintains control over his or her intake.

References

Acharyya, S., & Guttridge, D.C. (2007). Cancer cachexia signaling pathways continue to emerge yet much still points to the proteasome. *Clinical Cancer Research, 13,* 1356–1361.

American Medical Association. (2001). *AMA policy.* Retrieved June 1, 2007, from http://www .ama-assn.org

Barber, M.D., & Fearon, K.C. (2001). Tolerance and incorporation of a high-dose eicosapentaenoic acid diester emulsion by patients with pancreatic cancer cachexia. *Lipids, 36,* 347–351.

Barber, M.D., McMillan, D.C., Preston, T., Ross, J.A., & Fearon, K.C. (2000). Metabolic response to feeding in weight-losing pancreatic cancer patients and its modulation by a fish-oil-enriched nutritional supplement. *Clinical Science (Lond), 98,* 389–399.

Berenstein, E.G., & Ortiz, Z. (2005). Megestrol acetate for the treatment of anorexia-cachexia syndrome. *Cochrane Database of Systematic Reviews 2005,* Issue 2. Art. No.: CD004310. DOI: 10.1002/146518558. CD004310.pub2.

Bhogal, A.S., Lorite, M.L., & Tisdale, M.J. (2006). Changes in nucleic acid and protein levels in atrophying skeletal muscle in cancer cachexia. *Anticancer Research, 26,* 4149–4154.

Boughton, B. (2003). Drug increases lean tissue mass in patients with cancer. *Lancet Oncology, 4,* 135.

Bruera, E., Belzile, M., Neumann, C., Harsanyi, Z., Babul, N., & Darke, A. (2000). A double-blind, crossover study of controlled-release metoclopramide and placebo for the chronic nausea and dyspepsia of advanced cancer. *Journal of Pain and Symptom Management, 19,* 427–435.

Byock, I. (2000). Completing the continuum of care: Integrating life-prolongation and palliation. *CA: A Cancer Journal for Clinicians, 50,* 123–132.

Cannabis-In-Cachexia-Study-Group, Strasser, F., Luftner, D., Possinger, K., Ernst, G., Ruhstaller, T., et al. (2006). Comparison of orally administered cannabis extract and delta-9-tetrahydrocannabinol in treating patients with cancer-related anorexia-cachexia syndrome: A multicenter, phase III, randomized, double-blind, placebo-controlled clinical trial from the Cannabis-In-Cachexia-Study-Group. *Journal of Clinical Oncology, 24,* 3394–3400.

Del Fabbro, E., Dalal, S., & Bruera, E. (2006). Symptom control in palliative care—part II: Cachexia/Anorexia and fatigue. *Journal of Palliative Care, 9,* 409–420.

Dewey, A., Baughan, C., Dean, T., Higgins, B., & Johnson, I. (2007). Eicosapentaenoic acid (EPA, an omega-3 fatty acid from fish oils) for the treatment of cancer cachexia. *Cochrane Database of Systematic Reviews 2007,* Issue 1. Art. No.: CD004597. DOI: 10.1002/14651858. CD004597.pub2.

Fearon, K.C., Von Meyenfeldt, M.F., Moses, A.G., Van Geenen, R., Roy, A., Gouma, D.J., et al. (2003). Effect of a protein and energy dense N-3 fatty acid enriched oral supplement on loss of weight and lean tissue in cancer cachexia: A randomized double blind trial. *Gut, 52,* 1479–1486.

Fornari, A., & McCallum, P.D. (2006). Nutrition therapy in palliative care. In L. Elliott, L.L. Molseed, P.D. McCallum, & B. Grant (Eds.), *The clinical guide to oncology nutrition* (2nd ed., pp. 201–207). Chicago: American Dietetic Association.

Hoda, D., Jatoi, A., Burnes, J., Loprinzi, C., & Kelly, D. (2005). Should patients with advanced, incurable cancers ever be sent home with total parenteral nutrition? *Cancer, 103,* 863–868.

Hutton, J.L., Martin, L., Field, C.J., Wismer, W.V., Bruera, E.D., Watanabe, S.M., et al. (2006). Dietary patterns in patients with advanced cancer: Implications for anorexia-cachexia therapy. *American Journal of Clinical Nutrition, 84,* 1163–1170.

Isenring, E.A., Bauer, J.D., & Capra, S. (2007). Nutrition support using the American Dietetic Association medical nutrition therapy protocol for radiation oncology patients improves dietary intake compared with standard practice. *Journal of the American Dietetic Associaiton, 107,* 404–412.

Isenring, E.A., Capra, S., & Bauer, J.D. (2004a). Nutrition intervention is beneficial in oncology outpatients receiving radiotherapy to the gastrointestinal or head and neck area. *British Journal of Cancer, 91,* 447–452.

Isenring, E.A., Capra, S., & Bauer, J.D. (2004b). Patient satisfaction is rated higher by radiation oncology outpatients receiving nutrition intervention compared to usual care. *Journal of Human Nutrition and Dietetics, 17,* 145–152.

Kuroda, K., Nakashima, J., Kanao, K., Kikuchi, E., Miyajima, A., Horiguchi, Y., et al. (2007). Interleukin 6 is associated with cachexia in patients with prostate cancer. *Urology, 69,* 113–117.

Lundholm, K., Korner, U., Gunnebo, L., Sixt-Ammilon, P., Fouladiun, M., Daneryd, P., et al. (2007). Insulin treatment in cancer cachexia: Effects on survival, metabolism, and physical functioning. *Clinical Cancer Research, 13,* 2699–2706.

MacDonald, N. (2007). Cancer cachexia and targeting chronic inflammation: A unified approach to cancer treatment and palliative/supportive care. *Journal of Supportive Oncology, 5,* 157–162.

Marin Caro, M.M., Laviano, A., & Pichard, C. (2007). Nutritional intervention and quality of life in adult oncology patients. *Clinical Nutrition, 26,* 289–301.

Mateen, F., & Jatoi, A. (2006). Megestrol acetate for the palliation of anorexia in advanced, incurable cancer patients. *Clinical Nutrition, 25,* 711–715.

Melstrom, L.G., Melstrom, K.A., Jr., Ding, X.Z., & Adrian, T.E. (2007). Mechanisms of skeletal muscle degradation and its therapy in cancer cachexia. *Histology and Histopathology, 22,* 805–814.

Miller, F.G., Fins, J.J., & Snyder, L. (2000). Assisted suicide compared with refusal of treatment: A valid distinction? University of Pennsylvania Center for Bioethics Assisted Suicide Consensus Panel. *Annals of Internal Medicine, 132,* 470–475.

Moses, A.W., Slater, C., Preston, T., Barber, M.D., & Fearon, K.C. (2004). Reduced total energy expenditure and physical activity in cachectic patients with pancreatic cancer can be modulated by an energy and protein dense oral supplement enriched with n-3 fatty acids. *British Journal of Cancer, 90,* 996–1002.

National Comprehensive Cancer Network Nutrition Support Panel. (2006). *Practice guidelines in oncology—Palliative care.* Rockledge, PA: Author.

Odelli, C., Burgess, D., Bateman, L., Hughes, A., Ackland, S., Gillies, J., et al. (2005). Nutrition support improves patient outcomes, treatment tolerance and admission characteristics in esophageal cancer. *Clinical Oncology, 17,* 639–645.

Pascual, A., Roque, F.M., Urrutia, C.G., Berenstein, E.G., Almenar Pasies, B., Balcells Alegre, M., et al. (2004). Systematic review of megestrol acetate in the treatment of anorexia-cachexia syndrome. *Journal of Pain and Symptom Management, 27,* 360–369.

Quill, T.E., & Byock, I.R. (2000a). Responding to intractable terminal suffering. *Annals of Internal Medicine, 133,* 561–562.

Quill, T.E., & Byock, I.R. (2000b). Responding to intractable terminal suffering: The role of terminal sedation and voluntary refusal of food and fluids. *Annals of Internal Medicine, 132,* 408–414.

Ravasco, P., Monteiro-Grillo, I., Marques Vidal, P., & Camilo, M.E. (2005). Impact of nutrition on outcome: A prospective randomized controlled trial in patients with head and neck cancer undergoing radiotherapy. *Head and Neck, 27,* 659–668.

Shang, E., Weiss, C., Post, S., & Kachler, G. (2006). The influence of early supplementation of parenteral nutrition on quality of life and body composition in patients with advanced cancer. *Journal of Parenteral and Enteral Nutrition, 30,* 222–230.

Skipworth, R.J., Stewart, G.D., Dejong, C.H., Preston, T., & Fearon, K.C. (2007). Pathophysiology of cancer cachexia: Much more than host-tumour interaction? *Clinical Nutrition, 26,* 667–676.

Solvay Pharmaceuticals. (2006). Marinol [Package insert]. Retrieved June 1, 2007, from http://www .marinol.com.

Strasser, F., & Bruera, E.D. (2002). Update on anorexia and cachexia. *Hematology/Oncology Clinics of North America, 16,* 589–617.

Von Roenn, J.H. (2006). Pharmacologic management of nutrition impact symptoms associated with cancer. In L. Elliott, L.L. Molseed, P.D. McCallum, & B. Grant (Eds.), *The clinical guide to oncology nutrition* (2nd ed., pp. 201–207). Chicago: American Dietetic Association.

Von Roenn, J.H., Tchekmedyian, S., Sheng, K.N., & Ottery, F.D. (2002). Oxandrolone in cancer-related weight loss: Improvement in weight, body cell mass (BCM), performance status, and quality of life (QOL). *Proceedings of the American Society of Clinical Oncology, 363a,* Abstract 1450.

Walsh, D., Nelson, K.A., & Mahmoud, F.A. (2003). Established and potential therapeutic applications of cannabinoids in oncology. *Supportive Care in Cancer, 11,* 137–143.

Wilson, J., Plourde, J.Y., Marshall, D., Yoshida, S., Chow, W., Harsanyi, Z., et al. (2002). Long-term safety and clinical effectiveness of controlled-release metoclopramide in cancer-associated dyspepsia syndrome: A multicentre evaluation. *Journal of Palliative Care, 18,* 84–91.

Anxiety

Jennifer Fournier, RN, MSN, AOCN®, CHPN

Definition

Anxiety is a multifaceted, emotional response that vacillates along a continuum from a normal feeling of apprehension and fear to debilitating anxiety disorders, such as generalized anxiety disorder, panic disorder, post-traumatic stress disorder, social anxiety disorder, acute stress disorder, phobias, obsessive-compulsive disorder, or anxiety disorder caused by a medical condition (Heidrich & Esper, 2007; Kelly, McClement, & Chochinov, 2006; National Comprehensive Cancer Network [NCCN], 2007). Anxiety is the most common disorder seen in the general public as shown by the *National Comorbidity Survey* and the cause of significant social debility (Katon & Roy-Byrne, 2007). Anxiety is included in the top seven disorders in the *Diagnostic and Statistical Manual of Mental Disorders* (fourth edition), (DSM-IV) (NCCN). The four most frequent anxiety disorders seen in primary care are generalized anxiety disorder, social anxiety disorder, panic disorder, and post-traumatic stress disorder (Katon & Roy-Byrne; Kroenke, Spitzer, Williams, Monahan, & Lowe, 2007). The most frequently identified anxiety disorder in the palliative care setting is generalized anxiety disorder, followed closely by panic disorder (Wilson et al., 2007).

Anxiety is manifested in degrees, which can be described as mild, moderate, severe, and panic (Heidrich & Esper, 2007), and may have physical, emotional, psychosocial, and spiritual roots. Mild anxiety can be a stimulus to get something accomplished, whereas severe or continual anxiety can be physically or psychologically harmful.

Pathophysiology and Etiology

The human body is programmed to respond to potentially dangerous situations through the sympathetic branch of the autonomic nervous system evoking the fight-or-flight response. When this response is prolonged or occurs too frequently,

The author would like to acknowledge Pamela Spencer, BA, MSN, BSN, FNP, for her contribution that remains unchanged from the first edition.

problems ensue. Physical problems associated with excess anxiety in the palliative population can include hypertension, palpitations, hypercoagulation, hyperglycemia, nausea, and tissue destruction (Heidrich & Esper, 2007). Anxiety can be a risk factor for the development of Parkinson disease, as well as an early symptom of the disease (Ferreri, Agbokou, & Gauthier, 2006).

Assessment of anxiety includes subjective feelings, objective findings, and review of physical functions. The palliative care patient may describe feelings of apprehension, fear, anger, uneasiness, helplessness, nervousness, vulnerability, and changes in attention span. The observer may see fidgeting, tenseness, and trembling. Other physical characteristics include increased vital signs, dilated pupils, diaphoresis, dyspnea, pallor, flushing, dry mouth, nausea, and urinary frequency (Heidrich & Esper, 2007). Low systolic blood pressure has been linked to anxiety and depression in the older population (Hildrum et al., 2007).

Many patients experience some level of anxiety during the course of their illness. Although 14%–60% of patients experience a substantial degree of anxiety or distress (Katon & Roy-Byrne, 2007; Kelly et al., 2006; Kroenke et al., 2007; NCCN, 2007; Wilson et al., 2007), less than 10% of anxiety disorders are recognized and treated (NCCN). This can be attributed in part to the stigma associated with emotional issues. NCCN prefers the term *distress* to relate to any psychosocial disorders, including anxiety, because *distress* is more socially acceptable with less negative connotations.

Depression frequently is present in patients who are also experiencing anxiety. Increased symptom burden, existential suffering, and decreased functionality lead to a decreased quality of life for patients experiencing the comorbid conditions of anxiety and depression (Badger, Segrin, Dorros, Meek, & Lopez, 2007; Heidrich & Esper, 2007; Katon & Roy-Byrne, 2007; Kelly et al., 2006; Wilson et al., 2007). The *Canadian National Palliative Care Survey* reported that 66% of patients receiving palliative care who are identified as having anxiety also met DSM-IV criteria for depression and that 45% also met the DSM-IV criteria for an additional anxiety disorder. Other significant findings of this survey were that 83% of palliative care patients with anxiety and depression reported a moderate to extreme level of global suffering. These patients reported physical symptoms, social concerns, and existential issues; were younger; were more likely to be female; had smaller social networks; and were less active in organized religion (Wilson et al.).

Manifestations

- Restlessness
- Trembling
- Uneasiness
- Sweating
- Dilated pupils
- Dry mouth
- Urinary frequency
- Increased systolic blood pressure

- Tachypnea
- Tachycardia
- Dyspnea
- Dizziness
- Breathlessness
- Flushing
- Pallor
- Chest pain
- Abdominal pain
- Nausea and vomiting

(Ferreri et al., 2006; Heidrich & Esper, 2007)

General Management Principles

A. Pharmacologic interventions
1. Pharmacologic treatment of anxiety is suggested when anxiety is severe, limits quality of life, or is accompanied by depression. Antidepressants, selective serotonin reuptake inhibitors (SSRIs), and venlafaxine have shown efficacy for concomitant treatment of depression and anxiety. Anxiety with pronounced sympathetic symptoms, such as tremors and palpitations, may be treated with propranolol prior to the anxiety-provoking stimulus (National Guidelines Clearinghouse [NGC], 2003).
2. A substantial number of patients fail to respond to first-line medication interventions, and relapse is common (Ipser et al., 2006). Sustained remissions are more likely with long-term maintenance treatment of anxiety disorders following improvement of acute symptoms. Panic disorder and social phobia medications should be continued for six months, and medications for obsessive-compulsive disorder should be continued for one year. Discontinuation of anxiolytics should be done gradually and under careful supervision (NCCN, 2007). Patients taking antidepressants must be monitored for suicidal ideations (NGC, 2003).

B. Nonpharmacologic interventions
1. Psychotherapy with or without antidepressants and anxiolytics is the recommended first-line of treatment for anxiety (Kroenke et al., 2007; NGC, 2003). If the patient is not responsive to these treatment modalities, the psychotherapy should be reevaluated, in conjunction with a review of the medication. Additional support, education, and neuroleptics also may be necessary at this point. If the patient's condition remains unchanged, further evaluation is necessary to assess for other anxiety disorders (NGC). All patients should be screened for anxiety along the continuum of care, including at the initial visit, at routine intervals, with changes in disease status, and as clinically indicated. Canada has made emotional distress its sixth vital sign to be assessed routinely, but no minimum standards exist for psychosocial care in the United States (NCCN, 2007).

2. Cognitive behavioral therapy has the strongest support of all psychotherapies for the treatment of anxiety disorders (Ayers, Sorrell, Thorp, & Wetherell, 2007; Hill & Brettle, 2005; Hunot, Churchill, Teixeira, & Silva de Lima, 2006; Katon & Roy-Byrne, 2007; Kroenke et al., 2007). Cognitive behavioral therapy is equally effective in older and younger adults without the added burden of potential polypharmacy (Hill & Brettle). Separation anxiety can be seen in adults with panic disorder, which may begin in adulthood or be carried over from childhood and may respond to cognitive behavioral therapy (Harvard Mental Health Letter, 2007).

3. Exercise is likely to be effective in the treatment of anxiety (Badger et al., 2007; Saxena, van Ommeren, Tang, & Armstrong, 2005). Any type of exercise can be helpful and would be worthwhile for patients in the palliative care setting who are physically able to participate in an exercise regimen.

4. The current mental-health care system is challenged to meet the need for care of anxiety disorders. Paraprofessionals may have a role in the treatment of anxiety disorders, especially when compared to no treatment at all (den Boer, Wiersma, Russo, & van den Bosch, 2005). Collaborative care models, based on evidence-based practice utilizing paraprofessionals and allied healthcare professionals such as nurses, have been shown to be successful in managing depression (Katon & Roy-Byrne, 2007). These same models could likely be effective in assisting with the management of anxiety disorders as well, with clinicians as the key to initial identification of anxiety issues because of their unique role in patient care (Christie & Moore, 2004; NCCN, 2007). Telephone-delivered psychosocial interventions are another promising way to meet the needs of patients with anxiety disorders (Badger et al., 2007).

5. Complementary and alternative therapies are used by as many as 91% of patients with cancer (Stephenson, Swanson, Dalton, Keefe, & Engelke, 2007; Wyatt, Sikorskii, Siddiqi, & Given, 2007; Zick et al., 2006).

   a) Complementary therapies such as meditation, relaxation, reflexology, massage therapy with or without aromatherapy, guided imagery, humor, and virtual reality may have a role in anxiety management (Arias, Steinberg, Banga, & Trestman, 2006; Christie & Moore, 2004; Fellowes, Barnes, & Wilkinson, 2004; Krisanaprakornkit, Krisanaprakornkit, Piyavhatkul, & Laopaiboon, 2005; Lane, Seskevich, & Pieper, 2007; Roffe, Schmidt, & Ernst, 2005; Schneider & Hood, 2007; Wyatt et al., 2007). Reflexology was shown to have a significant effect on anxiety and may be taught to caregivers to be used with patients (Stephenson et al., 2007).

   b) Herbal therapies are included in complementary and alternative therapies. Essiac, a combination of at least four different herbs, consumed as a tea mostly by patients with breast cancer, was not shown to positively affect anxiety (Zick et al., 2006). Valerian is another herbal therapy that may not be effective for treating anxiety (Miyasaka, Atallah, & Soares, 2006). On the other hand, passiflora, or passionflower extract (Miyasaka et al.), and kava may have some benefit. Kava extract was the most promising herb in the treatment of anxiety (Pittler & Ernst, 2002), but its use poses a potential risk for hepatic toxicity or failure (Wasik, 2008).

Management

A. Death is not imminent.
1. **Level I—high level of evidence**
   (Arias et al., 2006; Heidrich & Esper, 2007; Hill & Brettle, 2005; Kapczinski, Lima, Souza, Cunha, & Schmitt, 2003; NCCN, 2007; NGC, 2003; Wasik, 2008)
   a) Cognitive behavioral therapy
      (1) Improvement seen in two-thirds of patients at six months
      (2) Shown to have the most consistent evidence of support
      (3) May increase efficacy of drug treatments
      (4) Useful in treatment of adults age 50 years and older
   b) SSRIs—First-line medication
      (1) Paroxetine (Paxil®) ($$$)—10–60 mg every morning; max 60 mg/day
         (a) Most studied
         (b) Few side effects
      (2) Sertraline (Zoloft®) ($$$)—start 25 mg po daily; max 200 mg/day
      (3) Fluoxetine (Prozac®) ($$$)—20–40 mg po every morning; max 80 mg/day
      (4) Citalopram (Celexa®) ($$$)—20 mg po daily; max 60 mg/day
         (a) Monitor for suicidal ideation.
         (b) Weigh risk versus benefit.
         (c) Avoid abrupt cessation.
   c) Antidepressants preferred over benzodiazepines
      (1) Clomipramine (Anafranil®) ($$$)—150–250 mg po at bedtime
         (a) Start 25 mg, increase gradually to effective dose.
         (b) Monitor for suicidal ideation.
      (2) Imipramine (Tofranil®) ($$$)—50 mg po daily; maximum 200 mg/day, 100 mg/day in older adults
         (a) Monitor for suicidal ideation.
         (b) Avoid abrupt cessation.
         (c) Monitor drug levels.
   d) Benzodiazepines
      (1) Alprazolam (Xanax®) ($)—0.25–0.5 mg po two to three times daily; max 2 mg/day in older adults
         (a) Short half-life (< 12 hours)
         (b) Multiple drug interactions
      (2) Lorazepam (Ativan®) ($$$)—0.5 mg po every six to eight hours; max 3 mg/day in older adults

        (a) Medium half-life of 10–20 hours

        (b) Preferred benzodiazepine with hepatic impairment

    (3) Diazepam (Valium®) ($)—2–10 mg po two to four times daily

        (a) Long half-life of 20–120 hours

        (b) Active metabolites

    (4) Clonazepam (Klonopin®) ($$)—start 0.25–0.5 mg po two to three times daily; max 4 mg/day

        (a) Half-life of 18–50 hours

        (b) Rapid relief

        (c) Monitor patient closely when discontinued.

  e) Serotonin norepinephrine reuptake inhibitors (SNRIs)

    (1) Venlafaxine (Effexor®) ($$$)—75–225 mg po daily

        (a) No anticholinergic, sedative, or orthostatic hypotension effects

        (b) Overdose more likely to be fatal

    (2) Trazodone ($)—50–100 mg po two or three times a day

        (a) Monitor for suicidal ideation.

        (b) Advise males of the possibility of priapism.

  f) Complementary therapies

    (1) Meditation

    (2) Relaxation

2. **Level II—moderate level of evidence**

(Chessick et al., 2006; Christie & Moore, 2004; Fellowes et al., 2004; NGC, 2003; Roffe et al., 2005; Saxena et al., 2005; Schneider & Hood, 2007; Stephenson et al., 2007; Wasik, 2008; Wyatt et al., 2007)

  a) Benzodiazepines

  b) Azapirone antidepressants

    (1) Imipramine (Tofranil) ($$$)—50–300 mg po at bedtime

        (a) May lower seizure threshold.

        (b) Monitor for suicidal ideation.

        (c) Weigh risk versus benefit.

    (2) Buspirone (BuSpar®) ($)—7.5–15 mg po bid daily

    (3) Benzodiazepines may be more effective and better accepted than azapirones in the treatment of anxiety; however, studies show conflicting evidence.

  c) Antidepressants

    (1) Nefazodone ($$$)—150–300 mg po bid; max 600 mg/day

        (a) Rarely, neuroleptic malignant syndrome may be seen.

        (b) Monitor for suicidal ideation.

        (c) Monitor liver function for possible hepatic failure.

    (2) Mirtazapine (Remeron®) ($$$)—15 mg at bedtime; max dose 45 mg

        (a) Make dose changes at one- to two-week intervals.

        (b) Monitor for suicidal ideation.

  d) Nonbenzodiazepine antianxiety agents

(1) Hydroxyzine (Vistaril®) ($)—50 mg po daily; may increase to four times daily; maximum 400 mg/day

(2) Promethazine—25–50 mg po, pr, IM, or IV every four to six hours, as needed

    (a) Monitor for respiratory depression.

    (b) Avoid use with other respiratory depressant–effect drugs.

  e) Beta-blockers

    (1) Propranolol (Inderal®) ($$)—10–40 mg po

      (a) Take 45–60 minutes prior to anxiety-provoking stimulus that produces pronounced sympathetic symptoms, such as tremors and palpitations.

      (b) Avoid abrupt cessation.

      (c) Taper gradually.

    (2) Atenolol (Tenormin®) ($$)—start 50 mg po daily

      (a) Avoid abrupt cessation.

      (b) Dose may be increased after seven days.

  f) Physical activity and exercise

  g) Complementary therapies

    (1) Reflexology (can be taught to caregivers)

    (2) Humor

    (3) Massage

      (a) Provides short-term benefit

      (b) Conflicting evidence regarding the addition of aromatherapy to massage

    (4) Guided imagery

    (5) Virtual reality

3. **Level III—low level of evidence**

  Herbal treatment (Miyasaka et al., 2006; Pittler & Ernst, 2002; Wasik, 2008)

  a) Passiflora (passionflower extract)—May be as effective as benzodiazepines

  b) Kava extract—Potential for hepatic toxicity or failure

B. Death is imminent.

  1. Treatment of anxiety should be continued as long as needed for the actively dying patient.

  2. Comfort measures should be continued or initiated as appropriate.

  3. Support should be available as needed.

  4. Overstimulation should be avoided.

Patient Outcomes

A. Anxiety is at an acceptable level.

B. Patient experiences restful sleep.

C. No physical manifestations of anxiety are present.

D. Comfort is maintained.

References

Arias, A.J., Steinberg, K., Banga, A., & Trestman, R.L. (2006). Systematic review of the efficacy of meditation techniques as treatments for medical illness. *Journal of Alternative and Complementary Medicine, 12,* 817–832.

Ayers, C.R., Sorrell, J.T., Thorp, S.R., & Wetherell, J.L. (2007). Evidence-based psychological treatments for late-life anxiety [Abstract]. *Psychology and Aging, 22,* 8–17.

Badger, T., Segrin, C., Dorros, S.M., Meek, P., & Lopez, A.M. (2007). Depression and anxiety in women with breast cancer and their partners. *Nursing Research, 56,* 44–53.

Chessick, C.A., Allen, M.H., Thase, M.E., Batista Miralha da Cunha, A.B.C., Kapczinski, F.F.K., de Lima, M.S.M.L., et al. (2006). Azapirones for generalized anxiety disorder. *Cochrane Database of Systematic Reviews 2006,* Issue 3. Art. No.: CD006115. DOI: 1002/14651858. CD006115.

Christie, W., & Moore, C. (2004). The impact of humor on patients with cancer. *Clinical Journal of Oncology Nursing, 9,* 211–218.

den Boer, P.C.A.M., Wiersma, D., Russo, S., & van den Bosch, R.J. (2005). Paraprofessionals for anxiety and depressive disorders. *Cochrane Database of Systematic Reviews 2005,* Issue 2. Art. No.: CD004688. DOI: 10.1002/14651858. CD004688.pub2.

Fellowes, D., Barnes, K., & Wilkinson, S. (2004). Aromatherapy and massage for symptom relief in patients with cancer. *Cochrane Database of Systematic Reviews 2004,* Issue 2. Art. No.: CD002287. DOI: 10.1002/14651858. CD002287.pub2.

Ferreri, F., Agbokou, C., & Gauthier, S. (2006). Recognition and management of neuropsychiatric complications in Parkinson's disease. *Canadian Medical Association Journal, 175,* 1545–1552.

Harvard Mental Health Letter. (2007, January). Separation anxiety. *Harvard Mental Health Letter, 23,* 1–3.

Heidrich, D.E., & Esper, P. (2007). Anxiety. In K.K. Kuebler, D.E. Heidrich, & P. Esper (Eds.), *Palliative and end-of-life care: Clinical practice guidelines* (2nd ed., pp. 245–257). St. Louis, MO: Elsevier Saunders.

Hildrum, B., Mykletun, A., Stordal, E., Bjelland, I., Dahl, A.A., & Holmen, J. (2007). Association of low blood pressure with anxiety and depression: The Nord-Trondelag health study. *Journal of Epidemiology and Community Health, 61,* 53–58.

Hill, A., & Brettle, A. (2005). The effectiveness of counselling with older people: Results of a systematic review. *Counselling and Psychotherapy Research, 5,* 265–272.

Hunot, V., Churchill, R., Teixeira, V., & Silva de Lima, M. (2007). Psychological therapies for generalized anxiety disorder. *Cochrane Database of Systematic Reviews 2007,* Issue 1. Art. No.: CD001848. DOI: 10.1002/14651858. CD001848.pub4.

Ipser, J.C., Carey, P., Dhansay, Y., Fakier, N., Seedat, S., & Stein, D.J. (2006). Pharmacotherapy augmentation strategies in treatment-resistant anxiety disorders. *Cochrane Database of Systematic Reviews 2006,* Issue 4. Art. No.: CD005473. DOI: 10.1002/14651858. CD005473.pub2.

Kapczinski, F., Lima, M.S., Souza, J.S., Cunha, A., & Schmitt, R. (2003). Antidepressants for generalized anxiety disorder. *Cochrane Database of Systematic Reviews 2002,* Issue 2. Art. No.: CD003592. DOI: 10.1002/14651858. CD003592.

Katon, W., & Roy-Byrne, P. (2007). Anxiety disorders: Efficient screening is the first step in improving outcomes [Editorial]. *Annals of Internal Medicine, 146,* 390–391.

Kelly, B., McClement, S., & Chochinov, H.M. (2006). Measurement of psychological distress in palliative care. *Palliative Medicine, 20,* 779–789.

Krisanaprakornkit, T., Krisanaprakornkit, W., Piyavhatkul, N., & Laopaiboon, M. (2007). Meditation therapy for anxiety disorders. *Cochrane Database of Systematic Reviews 2006,* Issue 1. Art. No.: CD004998. DOI: 10.1002/14651858. CD004998.pub2.

Kroenke, K., Spitzer, R.L., Williams, J.B.W., Monahan, P.O., & Lowe, B. (2007). Anxiety disorders in primary care: Prevalence, impairment, comorbidity, and detection. *Annals of Internal Medicine, 146,* 317–325.

Lane, J.D., Seskevich, J.E., & Pieper, C.F. (2007). Brief meditation training can improve perceived stress and negative mood. *Alternative Therapies, 13,* 38–44.

Miyasaka, L.S., Atallah, A.N., & Soares, B.G.O. (2007). Passiflora for anxiety disorder. *Cochrane Database of Systematic Reviews 2007,* Issue 1. Art. No.: CD004518. DOI: 10.1002/14651858. CD004518.pub2.

National Comprehensive Cancer Network. (2007). *NCCN clinical practice guidelines in oncology: Distress management, version 1.2007.* Retrieved May 22, 2007, from http://www.nccn.org/professionals/physician_gls/PDF/distress.pdf

National Guidelines Clearinghouse. (2003, November). *Anxiety disorders.* Retrieved May 3, 2007, from http://www.guideline.gov/summary/summary.aspx?doc_id=5293&nbr=003

Pittler, M.H., & Ernst, E. (2001). Kava extract versus placebo for treating anxiety. *Cochrane Database of Systematic Reviews 2001,* Issue 4. Art. No.: CD003383. DOI: 10.1002/14651858. CD003383.

Roffe, L., Schmidt, K., & Ernst, E. (2005). A systematic review of guided imagery as an adjuvant cancer therapy. *Psycho-Oncology, 14,* 607–617.

Saxena, S., van Ommeren, M., Tang, K.C., & Armstrong, T.P. (2005). Mental health benefits of physical activity. *Journal of Mental Health, 14,* 445–451.

Schneider, S.M., & Hood, L.E. (2007). Virtual reality: A distraction intervention for chemotherapy. *Oncology Nursing Forum, 34,* 39–46.

Stephenson, N.L.N., Swanson, M., Dalton, J., Keefe, F.J., & Engelke, M. (2007). Partner-delivered reflexology: Effects on cancer pain and anxiety. *Oncology Nursing Forum, 34,* 127–132.

Wasik, M. (2008). Anxiety. In F.J. Domino (Ed.), *The 5-minute clinical consult 2008* (16th ed., pp. 84–85). Philadelphia: Lippincott Williams & Wilkins.

Wilson, K.G., Chochinov, H.M., Skirko, M.G., Allard, P., Chary, S., Gagnon, P.R., et al. (2007). Depression and anxiety disorders in palliative cancer care. *Journal of Pain and Symptom Management, 33,* 118–129.

Wyatt, G., Sikorskii, A., Siddiqi, A., & Given, C.W. (2007). Feasibility of a reflexology and guided imagery intervention during chemotherapy: Results of a quasi-experimental study. *Oncology Nursing Forum, 34,* 635–642.

Zick, S.M., Sen, A., Feng, Y., Green, J., Olatunde, S., & Boon, H. (2006). Trial of Essiac to ascertain its effects in women with breast cancer (TEA-BC). *Journal of Alternative and Complementary Medicine, 12,* 971–980.

Ascites

Debra E. Heidrich, MSN, RN, ACHPN®, AOCN®

Definition

Ascites is the abnormal accumulation of fluid in the peritoneal cavity.

Pathophysiology and Etiology

The most common cause of ascites is liver disease, usually cirrhosis. Ascites associated with liver disease is caused by a combination of portal hypertension and sodium retention. Fibrosis in the liver interferes with hepatic venous outflow, leading to portal hypertension. Portal hypertension overloads lymphatic drainage and initiates activities that increase sodium retention (Lingappa, 2003; Wongcharatrawee & Garcia-Tsao, 2001). These factors also may contribute to ascites associated with congestive heart failure and nephrotic syndrome (Kichian & Bain, 2004).

About 10% of patients with ascites have a malignancy as the primary cause (Rosenberg, 2006). The mechanisms causing ascites associated with liver cancer may be the same as for liver disease (i.e., portal hypertension and sodium retention) (Kichian & Bain, 2004). Tumors that seed the peritoneum may release vascular endothelial growth factor (VEGF), which increases capillary permeability, thus allowing proteins to enter the peritoneal space. This increase in microvessel permeability is believed to be the main contributor to malignant ascites (Adam & Adam, 2004). In addition, tumors may directly obstruct lymphatic channels, causing chylous ascites (Kichian & Bain).

Manifestations

- Weight gain
- Increasing abdominal girth, often identified by a change in the way clothes fit
- Abdominal pressure, discomfort, or pain
- Anorexia, early satiety, nausea and vomiting, or indigestion
- Dyspnea and orthopnea
- Constipation
- Urinary frequency

- Edema of lower extremities and scrotum
- Skin of abdomen taut and shiny
- Shifting dullness on percussion of abdomen
- Fluid wave felt on examination of abdomen

(Heidrich, 2007; Kichian & Bains, 2004)

Management

A. Death is not imminent.
1. **Level I—high level of evidence**
   a) Sodium restriction and diuretics are first-line treatment for ascites caused by cirrhosis (Runyon, 2004). These interventions often are not effective for malignant ascites (unless portal hypertension is a contributing factor) and can deplete intravascular volume.
      (1) Restrict dietary intake of sodium to 2 g/day or less.
      (2) Initiate diuretic therapy using spironolactone ($) 100 mg po combined with furosemide 40 mg po. The dosages may be increased every three to five days, maintaining the 100 to 40 mg ratio; the maximum dose of spironolactone is 400 mg/day and of furosemide is 160 mg/day (Runyon, 2004; Sandhu & Sanyal, 2005; Zebrowski et al., 1999).
   b) Peritoneovenous shunt should be considered for patients with refractory ascites associated with cirrhosis who are not candidates for paracentesis, transplant, or transjugular intrahepatic portasystemic stent-shunt ($$$$) (Runyon, 2004). The role of these procedures in ascites related to malignancy is not clear.
   c) Patients with ascitic fluid polymorphonuclear (PMN) leukocyte counts > 250 cells/mm³ should receive empiric antibiotic therapy (e.g., cefotaxime 2 g every eight hours) ($$) (Runyon, 2004).
2. **Level II—moderate level of evidence**
   a) Fluid restriction is not necessary unless serum sodium is < 120 to 125 mmol/L (Runyon, 2004).
   b) Paracentesis ($$$) provides symptomatic relief from a tense abdomen (Runyon, 2004).
      (1) Up to 5 liters can be safely drained from the abdomen without replacement of albumin in patients with diuretic-resistant tense abdomens (Runyon, 2004; Stephenson & Gilbert, 2002).
      (2) If > 5 liters is removed in patients with portal hypertension-related ascites, albumin replacement ($$) is recommended at a dose of 8–10 g per liter of ascites removed (Runyon, 2004; Wongcharatrawee & Garcia-Tsao, 2001). The role of albumin replacement after large-volume paracentesis for malignancy-associated ascites is not clear.
      (3) If ascites is related to portal hypertension, paracentesis should be followed by diuretic therapy.

(4) Consider placement of a tunneled drainage catheter ($$$$) to allow intermittent drainage without repeat paracentesis in malignant ascites (Iyengar & Herzog, 2002; Rosenberg, Courtney, Nemcek, & Omary, 2004).

c) Intracavitary chemotherapy ($$$–$$$$) may control ascites in patients whose tumors initially responded to systemic therapy, especially in patients with ascites related to ovarian or breast cancer (Adam & Adam, 2004).

d) Patients with ascitic fluid PMN counts < 250 cells/mm^3 and who have fever or abdominal pain or tenderness should receive empiric antibiotic therapy ($$) while awaiting results of cultures (Runyon, 2004).

3. **Level III—low level of evidence**
   a) Pharmacologic interventions
      (1) Analgesics ($–$$) for comfort.
      (2) Octreotide (Sandostatin®) ($$$)—Subcutaneous administration of 200–400 mcg/day has been reported to be effective in some cases of intractable ascites. The true cost-benefit ratio of this intervention has not been adequately evaluated (Cairns & Malone, 1999; Mincher, Evans, Jenner, & Varney, 2005; Waller & Caroline, 2000).
      (3) Anti-VEGF antibodies, anti-VEGF receptor antibodies, tumor necrosis factor, metalloproteinase inhibitors, interleukin-2, and beta-interferon are in phase I and II trials for treatment of malignant ascites (Adam & Adam, 2004; Numnum, Rocconi, Whitworth, & Barnes, 2006).
   b) Nonpharmacologic interventions (Heidrich, 2007; Kichian & Bain, 2004)
      (1) Elevate head of bed.
      (2) Encourage small, frequent meals and increase protein.
      (3) Employ measures to prevent constipation and to maintain bowel function.
      (4) Encourage the patient to wear loose-fitting clothing.
      (5) Elevate lower extremities when sitting.
      (6) Encourage meticulous skin care.
      (7) Place indwelling Foley catheter for urinary retention.

B. Death is imminent.
   1. Position for comfort.
   2. Discontinue any sodium or fluid restrictions.
   3. Continue to remove abdominal fluid via paracentesis if this promotes comfort for the patient.
      a) If a catheter has been placed for drainage of abdominal fluid, the cost and discomfort associated with the procedure is minimal and can greatly enhance comfort.
      b) If needle puncture is required, the discomfort associated with the procedure must be weighed against the potential increase in comfort

following the procedure. In addition, in the event that arrangements cannot be made to perform this procedure at the patient's current location, the physical, emotional, and financial burdens of transporting the patient to a clinic or hospital must be evaluated.

Patient Outcomes

A. Relief of abdominal discomfort is provided.

B. Dyspnea and orthopnea are relieved.

C. Ascites is controlled.

D. Regular bowel movements are present.

References

Adam, R.A., & Adam, Y.G. (2004). Malignant ascites: Past, present, and future. *Journal of the American College of Surgeons, 198,* 999–1011.

Cairns, W., & Malone, R. (1999). Octreotide as an agent for the relief of malignant ascites in palliative care patients. *Palliative Medicine, 19,* 429–430.

Heidrich, D. (2007). Ascites. In K.K. Kuebler, D.E. Heidrich, & P. Esper (Eds.), *Palliative and end-of-life care: Clinical practice guidelines* (2nd ed., pp. 259–268). St. Louis, MO: Elsevier Saunders.

Iyengar, T.D., & Herzog, R.J. (2002). Management of symptomatic ascites in recurrent ovarian cancer patients using an intra-abdominal semi-permanent catheter. *American Journal of Hospice and Palliative Care, 19,* 35–38.

Kichian, K., & Bain, V.G. (2004). Jaundice, ascites, and hepatic encephalopathy. In D. Doyle, G. Hanks, H. Cherny, & K. Calman (Eds.), *Oxford textbook of palliative medicine* (3rd ed., pp. 507–520). New York: Oxford University Press.

Lingappa, V.R. (2003). Liver disease. In S.J. McPhee, V.R. Lingappa, & W.F. Ganong (Eds.), *Pathophysiology of disease: An introduction to clinical medicine* (4th ed., pp. 380–419). New York: Lange Medical Books/McGraw-Hill.

Mincher, L., Evans, J., Jenner, M.W., & Varney, V.A. (2005). The successful treatment of chylous effusions in malignant disease with octreotide. *Clinical Oncology (Royal College of Radiology), 17,* 118–121.

Numnum, T.M., Rocconi, P., Whitworth, J., & Barnes, M.N. (2006). The use of bevacizumab to palliate symptomatic ascites in patients with refractory ovarian cancer. *Gynecologic Oncology, 102,* 425–428.

Rosenberg, S.M. (2006). Palliation of malignant ascites. *Gastroenterology Clinics of North America, 35,* 189–199.

Rosenberg, S., Courtney, A., Nemcek, A.A., Jr., & Omary, R.A. (2004). Comparison of percutaneous management techniques for recurrent malignant ascites. *Journal of Vascular Interventional Radiology, 15,* 1129–1131.

Runyon, B.A. (2004). AASLD practice guideline: Management of adult patients with ascites due to cirrhosis. *Hepatology, 39,* 841–856.

Sandhu, B.S., & Sanyal, A.J. (2005). Management of ascites in cirrhosis. *Clinics in Liver Disease, 9,* 715–732.

Stephenson, J., & Gilbert, J. (2002). The development of clinical guidelines on paracentesis for ascites related to malignancy. *Palliative Medicine, 16,* 213–218.

Waller, A., & Caroline, N.L. (2000). *Handbook of palliative care in cancer* (2nd ed.). Boston: Butter-worth-Heinemann.

Wongcharatrawee, S., & Garcia-Tsao, G. (2001). Clinical management of ascites and its complications. *Clinics in Liver Disease, 5,* 833–850.

Zebrowski, B.K., Liu, W., Ramirez, K., Akagi, Y., Mills, G.B., & Ellis, L.M. (1999). Markedly elevated levels of vascular endothelial growth factor in malignant ascites. *Annals of Surgical Oncology, 6,* 373–378.

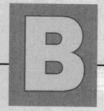

Bleeding

Bowel Obstruction

Bleeding

Ruth Canty Gholz, RN, MS, AOCN®

Definition

Bleeding is the loss of blood from the circulatory system.

Pathophysiology and Etiology

Bleeding can result from local vessel injury, disruption of a localized pathologic process, or a disorder of the hemostatic process. In the palliative care arena, bleeding occurs in approximately 6%–10% of patients (Prommer, 2005). It can be characterized as chronic, persistent, or acute. Bleeding may be slow, oozing, or rapid as in hemorrhage. Bleeding is very distressing to the patient and family and disturbs quality of life.

Assessment of bleeding is essential: A patient with massive bleeding is at risk for exsanguination.

Individuals at risk for bleeding are those with
- Thrombocytopenia or platelet dysfunction
- Coagulation deficits
- Fungating wounds
- Tumors on or surrounding blood vessels
- Liver failure
- Vascular malformations
- Friable tissue
- Portal hypertension
- Renal failure
- Brain metastases.

Manifestations

- Anemia
- Bleeding wounds or lesions
- Purpura
- Epistaxis

- Petechiae
- Coffee-ground emesis
- Frank blood loss
- Tachycardia
- Hemorrhage
- Hypotension
- Ecchymoses
- Shortness of breath
- Hematoma
- Restlessness
- Hemoptysis
- Sudden change in vision; severe headache
- Melena
- Vaginal bleeding
- Hematemesis
- Anxiety
- Hematuria
- Pallor

Management

A. General measures
   1. Prophylaxis is preferred (e.g., oral care, skin care, wound management, platelet transfusion) (Schiffer et al., 2001).
   2. Discuss wishes of the patient and palliative care goals.
   3. Identify source and cause (e.g., capillary, large vessel injury, disruption in coagulation) and control bleeding.
   4. If the patient is symptomatic and symptoms are reducing quality of life, perform hematologic workup, such as complete blood count, bleeding time, prothrombin time, international normalized ratio, fibrinogen, and D-dimer, to identify a reversible condition.

B. Palliative blood products ($$): If bleeding is causing distress or if administration of products would improve function and quality of life
   1. Platelets (Stanworth et al., 2004)
   2. Fresh frozen plasma
   3. Cryoprecipitate

C. Systemic management
   Level II—moderate level of evidence
   (Pereira & Phan, 2004)
   1. Antifibrinolytic agents
   2. Somatostatin
   3. Vasopressin
   4. Vitamin K (Back, 2001)

5. If patient *is* on anticoagulation, convert from warfarin to low-molecular-weight heparin ($$$).

D. Wounds
   1. **Level I—high level of evidence** ($$)
      (Prommer, 2005)
      a) Nonadherent dressings
      b) Pressure
      c) Packing
      d) Hemostatic dressing (e.g., absorbable collagen, fibrin sealants, alginates, oxidized cellulose and regenerated cellulose)
      e) Hemostatic agents (e.g., formalin, silver nitrate, sucralfate, acetone, epinephrine)
      f) QR Powder® for nosebleeds and malignant wounds
   2. See Skin Lesions.

E. Miscellaneous
   Level I—high level of evidence ($$)
   (Prommer, 2005)
   1. YAG laser for endobronchial lesions (Hain, Prasetvo, & Wright, 2007)
   2. Administer palliative radiation to establish a thrombosis.
   3. Perform transcatheter arterial embolization.
   4. Perform sclerotherapy procedure.
   5. Perform endoscopy utilizing electrocoagulation probes, epinephrine injection, microwaves, lasers, and argon plasma coagulation only after vasoconstrictor drugs have failed (Pereirra & Phan, 2004).
   6. Manage arterial rupture resulting in exsanguination.
      a) Prepare patient and family for possibility: primarily from head and neck cancers and centrally located lung cancers.
      b) Have dark towels at the bedside.
      c) Position patient on the side where the bleed would be the lowest.
      d) Sedate patient to reduce emotional distress of rupture.
      e) Provide emotional support.

Patient Outcomes

A. Bleeding is prevented or controlled when possible.

B. Patient comfort is maintained when bleeding cannot be controlled.

C. Patient and caregivers receive psychological support when exsanguination is inevitable.

References

Back, I.N. (2001). *Palliative medicine handbook.* Retrieved May 30, 2007, from http://book.pallcare .info/inderx.php?tid=78

Han, C.C., Prasetvo, D., & Wright, G.M. (2007). Endobronchial palliation using Nd: YAG laser is associated with improved survival when combined with multimodal adjuvant treatments. *Journal of Thoracic Oncology, 2,* 59–64.

Pereira J., & Phan, T. (2004). Management of bleeding in patients with advanced cancer. *Oncologist, 9,* 561–570.

Prommer, E. (2005). Management of bleeding in the terminally ill patient. *Hematology, 10,* 167–175.

Schiffer, C.A., Anderson, K.C., Bennett, C.L., Bernstein, S., Elting, L.S., Goldsmith, M., et al. (2001). Platelet transfusion for patients with cancer: Clinical practice guidelines of the American Society of Clinical Oncology. *Journal of Clinical Oncology, 19,* 1519–1538.

Stanworth, S.J., Hyde, C., Heddle, N., Rebulla, P., Brunskill, S., & Murphy, M.F. (2004). Prophylactic platelet transfusion for haemorrhage after chemotherapy and stem cell transplantation. *Cochrane Database of Systematic Reviews 2004,* Issue 4. Art. No.: CD004269. DOI: 10.1002/14651858. CD004269.pub2.

Bowel Obstruction

Pamela Spencer, BA, MSN, BSN, FNP

Definition

Bowel obstruction is defined as an occlusion of the lumen that prevents the propulsion of the intestinal contents from passing distally (Ripamonti & Mercadante, 2004). Therefore, with obstruction, the motor activities of the small intestine and/or colon become impaired (Hasler, 2003). Bowel obstruction is a consequence of a variety of conditions that include extrinsic, intrinsic, and intraluminal lesions (Yamada et al., 2005). Malignant bowel obstruction is a well-recognized complication in patients with advanced cancer who have abdominal and pelvic malignancies (Ripamonti & Mercadante). Bowel obstruction in the palliative care patient is a relatively frequent complication and may present acutely, but more commonly it is gradual in onset, intermittent, and variable in severity (Chilton & Faull, 2005). Any site in the bowel can be affected, from the gastroduodenal junction to the rectum and anus.

Pathophysiology and Etiology

Partial or complete obstruction often is multifactorial. An obstruction of the bowel can occur at any level and can be functional, mechanical, or both. Bowel obstruction occurs when the forward flow of gastric and intestinal contents through the gastrointestinal tract is blocked (Low, Chen, & Barone, 2003). With obstruction, the motor activities of the small intestine and/or colon are characterized by contractile patterns that serve the requirements of each organ that become impaired (Hasler, 2003). Malignant gastrointestinal obstruction occurs most commonly in patients with advanced abdominal or pelvic cancers: in 25% of patients with primary bowel cancer, 6% of patients with a primary ovarian cancer, and in about 40% of patients with advanced ovarian cancer (Chilton & Faull, 2005). Nonmalignant causes of bowel obstruction include adhesions from previous surgeries, incarcerated or strangulated hernias, pseudo-obstruction, and fecal impaction (Heidrich & Spencer, 2007).

Manifestations

The level of obstruction determines the different patterns of symptoms. The progression may be slow or fast, and from partial obstruction to complete occlu-

sion. Each level produces a different spectrum of symptoms differing in intensity of suffering.
- Obstruction in the proximal bowel can cause vomiting, severe dehydration, and electrolyte disturbances but with minimal abdominal distention.
- Blockage in the distal colon causes a large amount of fluid to accumulate in the bowel with third-spacing of fluids, dehydration, abdominal distention, and feculent vomiting.
- Abdominal pain is present in about 90% of patients presenting with a bowel obstruction.
- Nausea and vomiting occurs in 100% of patients with complete obstruction.
- Increased bowel sounds include classically tinkling noises, but these may be absent.
- Visible peristalsis is frequently present.

(Hirst & Regnard, 2003; Ripamonti & Mercadante, 2004)

Management

A. Death is not imminent.
   Level I—high level of evidence
   (Hirst & Regnard, 2003; Mercadante, Ferrera, Villari, & Marrazzo, 2004; Ripamonti & Mercadante, 2004; Smothers et al., 2003)
   1. Nasogastric intubation and fluid replacement ($$) can be used temporarily.
   2. Pharmacologic interventions
      a) Antiemetics ($)
         (1) Metoclopramide (Reglan®)—10 mg po every four to six hours or 40–60 mg over a 24-hour SC infusion
         (2) Haloperidol—5–15 mg/day SC
         (3) Prochlorperazine—25 mg po every eight hours, as needed
         (4) Chlorpromazine—50–100 mg po every eight hours, as needed
      b) Analgesics ($–$$$)—Opiate therapy as needed for relief of pain
      c) Anticholinergics ($)—Scopolamine hydrobromide—0.4 mg SC every four to six hours or 0.6–1.2 mg over a 24-hour SC infusion
      d) Somatostatin analog ($$$$)—Octreotide (Sandostatin®)—0.1 mg SC or 0.2–0.3 mg over a 24-hour SC infusion
      e) Corticosteroids ($)—Dexamethasone—8–16 mg po/SC daily
   3. Surgical interventions ($$–$$$$) should be considered in acute or complete obstruction, peritonitis, strangulated hernia, or gastric outlet obstruction.

B. Death is imminent.
   1. **Level I—high level of evidence**
      a) Manual removal of fecal impaction ($), various enemas
      b) Pharmacologic interventions
         (1) Stool softener ($)—Docusate sodium (Colace®)

      (2) Dexamethasone ($)—20 mg SC bid for 24 hours, then taper to lowest effective dose for reduction of symptoms

      (3) Hyoscyamine butylbromide (Levsin®) ($)—10–20 mg SC every four hours (every hour, as needed)

      (4) Octreotide (Sandostatin) ($$$)—50–100 mcg SC bid

  c) Insert nasogastric tube ($) for decompression and pain control.

  d) Stenting ($$$$) (Hirst & Regnard 2003; Mittal, Windsor, Woodfield, Casey, & Lane, 2004)

2. **Level II—moderate level of evidence**

  a) Provide appropriate mouth care (Hallenbeck, 2003).

  b) Psychosocial interventions (Bresalier, 2003).

Patient Outcomes

A. Regular bowel movements are maintained, if possible. If unable, manage symptoms of pain, nausea, and vomiting appropriately.

B. Respiratory system compromise is assessed, as secondary abdominal distention can occur.

C. Optimal comfort is maintained.

References

Bresalier, R.S. (2003). Malignant and premalignant lesions of the colon. In S.L. Friedman, K.R. McQuaid, & J.H. Grendell (Eds.), *Current diagnosis and treatment in gastroenterology* (2nd ed., pp. 407–435). New York: McGraw-Hill.

Chilton, A., & Faull, C. (2005). The management of gastrointestinal symptoms and advance liver disease. In C. Faull, Y. Carter, & L. Daniels (Eds.), *Handbook of palliative care* (2nd ed., pp. 150–185). Malden, MA: Blackwell Publishing.

Hallenbeck, J. (2003). *Palliative care perspectives.* New York: Oxford University Press.

Hasler, W.L. (2003). Motility of the small intestine and colon. In T. Yamada, D.H. Alpers, N. Kaplowitz, L. Laine, C. Owyang, & D.W. Powell (Eds.), *The textbook of gastroenterology* (4th ed., pp. 220–247). Philadelphia: Lippincott Williams & Wilkins.

Heidrich, D., & Spencer, P. (2007). Bowel obstruction. In K.K. Kuebler, D.E. Heidrich, & P. Esper (Eds.), *Palliative and end-of-life care: Clinical practice guidelines* (2nd ed., pp. 269–286). St. Louis, MO: Elsevier Saunders.

Hirst, B., & Regnard, C. (2003). Management of intestinal obstruction in malignant disease. *Clinical Medicine, 3,* 311–314.

Low, R.N., Chen, S.C., & Barone, R. (2003). Distinguishing benign from malignant bowel obstruction in patients with malignancy: Findings at MR imaging. *Radiology, 228,* 157–165.

Mercadante, S., Ferrera, P., Villari, P., & Marrazzo, A. (2004). Aggressive pharmacological treatment for reversing malignant bowel obstruction. *Journal of Pain and Symptom Management, 28,* 412–416.

Mittal, A., Windsor, J., Woodfield, J., Casey, P., & Lane, M. (2004). Matched study of three methods for palliation of malignant obstruction. *British Journal of Surgery, 91,* 205–209.

Ripamonti, C., & Mercadante, S. (2004). Pathophysiology and management of malignant bowel obstruction. In D. Doyle, G. Hanks, & N. Cherny (Eds.), *Oxford textbook of palliative medicine* (3rd ed., pp. 498–505). New York: Oxford University Press.

Smothers, L., Hynan, L., Fleming, J., Turnage, R., Simmang, C., & Anthony, T. (2003). Emergency surgery for colon carcinoma. *Diseases of the Colon and Rectum, 46,* 24–30.

Yamada, T., Alpers, D.H., Loren, L., Kaplowitz, N., Owyang, C., & Powell, D.W. (2005). Approach to the patient with ileus or obstruction. In T. Yamada, W.L. Hasler, J.M. Inadomi, M.A. Anderson, & R.S. Brown, Jr. (Eds.), *Handbook of gastroenterology* (2nd ed., pp. 94–100). Philadelphia: Lippincott Williams & Wilkins.

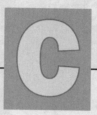

Caregiver Issues

Complementary and Alternative
Medicine and Integrative Medicine

Constipation

Cough

Cultural Competence

Caregiver Issues

Crystal Dea Moore, MA, PhD, MSW, MA

Definition

A recent national survey found that 21% of the adult population 18 years of age and older provide unpaid care to an adult family member or friend (National Alliance for Caregiving [NAC] & AARP, 2004). In this study, *caregiving* was defined as unpaid care to a relative or friend that included help with personal needs or household chores. A previous national study commissioned by AARP found that 19% of adults responded affirmatively when asked simply if they were "caregivers" (AARP, 2001). An additional 15% of respondents in this same study did not identify with the label "caregiver" but did indicate that they provided unpaid help (explicitly defined in terms of specific caregiving activities) to a relative or friend who had a disability or chronic illness.

Specific Issues in Palliative Care

A. Although the typical caregiver is a woman in her mid-forties with some college education who provides in excess of 20 hours of care each week to her mother, family caregivers are an increasingly diverse group. Sixty-one percent of caregivers are women, and 39% are men (NAC & AARP, 2004). The majority of family caregivers, male or female, fulfill multiple roles that include spouse, parent, and member of the workforce. A majority of family caregivers are employed outside the home. Three in 10 family caregivers help to care for more than one person.

B. Seventy-nine percent of family caregivers provide care to someone older than age 50, and the remaining 21% provide care to someone between the ages of 18 and 49. Caregivers of younger individuals are more likely to experience financial hardship as a result of their caregiving responsibilities (NAC & AARP, 2004).

The author would like to acknowledge Jerre Cory, MA, CSW, and Kim K. Kuebler, MN, RN, APRN-BC, for their contributions that remain unchanged from the first edition of this textbook.

C. The intensity of caregiving responsibilities and concomitant burden experienced among family caregivers varies. The NAC/AARP study (2004) found that the level of burden (measured by intensity of caregiving responsibilities), the perception of choice in taking on caregiver responsibilities, and the caregiver's own health status have the biggest impact on caregivers' perceived emotional stress, physical strain, or financial hardship.

D. Financial concerns can complicate family caregiving. As compared to Whites, Latino and African American family caregivers are at higher risk for financial hardship as a result of caregiving responsibilities because of various socioeconomic factors, including income and level of education (NAC & AARP, 2004).

E. Americans are living longer, thus increasing the demands on family caregivers. People who are living longer with advanced illness may be pushing the capacities of family caregivers to the limit. Most of these patients experience functional limitations that cause them to require daily assistance when performing routine activities.

F. Family caregivers need additional support, and unmet needs exist (NAC & AARP, 2004).
   1. Less than half of caregivers (48%) use outside services such as Meals-on-Wheels, formal respite, and adult day care. Use of unpaid services is more common than reliance on formal service providers.
   2. Two-thirds of caregivers indicate they have unmet needs related to providing care for their care recipient.
   3. One in five caregivers report they need help in talking with doctors and other medical providers and in making end-of-life decisions.
   4. Many caregivers cope with the emotional strains of caregiving through prayer (73%), seeking social support from friends or relatives (61%), and reading information about caregiving in books or on the Internet (44%).

G. Family caregivers often help patients to use and understand health-related information and provide patient support before, during, and after medical encounters (Glasser, Prohaska, & Gravdal, 2001; Silliman, Bhatti, Khan, Dukes, & Sullivan, 1996).

Strategies to Promote Effective Caregiver Involvement in Palliative Care

A. Given the importance of family caregivers for patient care, providers should make deliberate and intentional efforts to include them in ongoing discussions about patient care and treatment plans. Caregivers should be viewed as an integral and valued part of the healthcare team and treated with respect and consideration.

B. Ongoing assessment of patient and family caregiver needs should be a priority.
   1. As the patient's illness progresses, particularly when a substantive change in patient health status occurs, providers should discuss with the patient and family the preferred and most appropriate location and setting for continued care. Although many patients want to remain in their home, not all do, and as caregiving demands increase, this may not be a feasible option. Ongoing and open dialogue about the site of care should be maintained throughout the disease trajectory.
   2. Depression is common among family caregivers, and providers should pay attention to the mental health status of family caregivers. Without attention to caregivers' emotional and physical needs, the care of patients may suffer.
   3. Caregivers who are older or have their own health issues need to be made aware of the physical, emotional, and social demands that occur when choosing to care for a patient at home. Providers can help family caregivers to evaluate realistic expectations regarding care plans.

C. Providers should be aware of cultural issues that may affect the caregiving experience. For some groups, extended kin networks are available to help the primary caregiver, or caregiving demands may be increased because of multiple caregiving responsibilities. As previously indicated, some groups may be at higher risk for financial complications related to caregiving responsibilities.

D. Raising awareness about and connecting family caregivers to community resources can help to alleviate caregiver burden and promote positive outcomes for the family caregiver and patient.
   1. For caregivers of older patients, local agencies on aging can provide useful information and connections to community resources for older adults. Local contact numbers can be obtained by calling the Eldercare Locator, a free national service sponsored by the U.S. Administration on Aging, at 800-677-1116 or by visiting the national Web site at www.eldercare.gov.
   2. Hospice care is an option for patients of any age that have a prognosis of less than six months to live. Hospice care, a family-centered approach to end-of-life care, provides numerous caregiver resources, including in-home and respite care.
   3. Some states participate in the Medicaid Waiver Program, which is considered a "nursing home without walls." This program offers comprehensive formal caregiving in the home to people with limited financial resources.
   4. Caregivers also can be referred to Web-based resources such as the National Family Caregivers Association (NFCA), which seeks to educate, support, empower, and speak up for the more than 50 million Americans who care for those with a chronic illness or disability or the frailties of old age. NFCA reaches across the boundaries of diagnoses, relationships, and life stages to address the common needs and concerns of all family caregivers.

Its Web site is www.thefamilycaregiver.org and toll-free telephone number is 800-896-3650.

Evaluating the Evidence

A. Although few randomized controlled studies are performed to evaluate the effectiveness of interventions aimed at promoting positive outcomes for family caregivers, the literature in this area is increasing. For example, one randomized controlled study, which evaluated the effectiveness of a telephone support group for adult children and spouse caregivers of frail older adults, found that the intervention was more effective than usual care in reducing burden, depression, and pressing problems and in increasing knowledge and use of community services. However, no significant differences were found for spouse caregivers (Smith & Toseland, 2006).

B. One meta-analysis examining the effectiveness of caregiver interventions concluded that "interventions are, on average, successful in alleviating burden and depression, increasing general subjective well-being, and increasing caregiving ability/knowledge" (Sorensen, Pinquart, & Dubenstein, 2002, p. 369). Although many of the studies reviewed did not employ random assignment, the authors indicated that caregiver interventions have both broad and specific effects on outcomes.

C. According to a recent Cochrane review (Lee & Cameron, 2007), three randomized controlled trials provided no evidence of any benefit of respite care for older patients with dementia or their family caregivers, including outcomes related to caregiver burden. However, the reviewers indicated that "a host of methodological problems in available trials were identified."

Patient and Caregiver Outcomes

A. Caregivers who are supported in their caregiving responsibilities can maintain optimal well-being and recognize the physical, emotional, and social challenges that result from caregiving demands.

B. Evidence suggests that family caregivers can and do influence treatment plan implementation and adherence (Beals, Wight, Aneshensel, Murphy, & Miller-Martinez, 2006; Guberman, Lavoie, Pepin, Lauzon, & Montejo, 2006; Silliman et al., 1996; Vivian & Wilcox, 2000). One recent longitudinal survey study that involved both patients and family caregivers found that frequent, high-quality communication among family caregivers and healthcare professionals was related to caregivers' preparation to provide and manage patient care. This preparation and management led to improved patient outcomes, including better pain management, functional status, and mental health 12 weeks following knee surgery (Weinberg, Lusenhop, Gittell, & Kautz, 2007).

References

AARP. (2001). *Caregiver identification study*. Washington, DC: Author.

Beals, K.P., Wight, R.G., Aneshensel, C.S., Murphy, D.A., & Miller-Martinez, D. (2006). The role of family caregivers in HIV medication adherence. *AIDS Care, 18,* 589–596.

Glasser, M., Prohaska, T.R., & Gravdal, J. (2001). Elderly patients and their accompanying caregivers on medical visits. *Research on Aging, 23,* 326–348.

Guberman, N., Lavoie, J.P., Pepin, J., Lauzon, S., & Montejo, M.E. (2006). Formal service practitioners' views of family caregivers' responsibilities and difficulties. *Canadian Journal of Aging, 25,* 43–53.

Lee, H., & Cameron, M. (2007). Respite care for people with dementia and their carers. *Cochrane Database of Systematic Reviews 2004,* Issue 2. Art. No.: CD004396. DOI: 10.1002/14651858. CD004396.pub2.

National Alliance for Caregiving & AARP. (2004). *Caregiving in the U.S.* Washington, DC: Authors.

Silliman, R.A., Bhatti, S., Khan, A., Dukes, K.A., & Sullivan, L.M. (1996). The care of older persons with diabetes mellitus: Families and primary care physicians. *Journal of the American Geriatrics Society, 44,* 1314–1321.

Smith, T., & Toseland, R. (2006). Effectiveness of a telephone support group for frail older adults. *Gerontologist, 46,* 620–629.

Sorensen, S., Pinquart, M., & Dubenstein, P. (2002). How effective are interventions with caregivers? An updated meta-analysis. *Gerontologist, 42,* 356–372.

Vivian, B.G., & Wilcox, J.R. (2000). Compliance communication in home health care: A mutually reciprocal process. *Qualitative Health Research, 10,* 103–116.

Weinberg, D., Lusenhop, R., Gittell, J., & Kautz, C. (2007). Coordination between formal providers and informal caregivers. *Health Care Management Review, 32,* 140–149.

Complementary and Alternative Medicine and Integrative Medicine

Georgia M. Decker, MS, APRN-BC, CN®, AOCN®

Definition

Complementary and alternative medicine (CAM) is often defined in several ways. The term *alternative* has been used as an umbrella term to describe therapies not taught in medical schools or hospitals in the United States. This definition is no longer accurate because many medical schools include these therapies in their curricula, and some are provided to patients in a variety of settings (Eisenberg et al., 1993). The interchangeable use of the terms *complementary* and *alternative* has led to miscommunication and misunderstandings among clinicians, the public, and patients because *complementary* and *alternative* are not the same. A therapy is defined by the intent with which it is used; therefore, *alternative* refers to therapies employed instead of conventional therapy, and *complementary* refers to therapies that supplement conventional therapy. The more current terms *integrative* or *integrated* are preferred because they reflect the use of CAM therapies in combination with conventional treatments (Oncology Nursing Society, 2006). Using an integrated framework provides an opportunity to incorporate these therapies safely and appropriately.

Multiple approaches to categorizing CAM exist. Currently, the National Center for Complementary and Alternative Medicine (NCCAM) classifies CAM therapies into five domains:
- Alternative medical systems
- Mind-body interventions
- Biologically based therapies
- Manipulative and body-based methods
- Energy therapies.

The National Cancer Institute (NCI, 2004a) Office of Cancer Complementary and Alternative Medicine (OCCAM) expanded the NCCAM domains by adding categories for clarification: movement therapy and pharmacologic and biologic treatments with a subcategory of complex natural products (NCI, 2004b). Table 9-1 provides definitions and examples of these domains.

The author would like to acknowledge Nancy K. English, RN, PhD, APN, CS, for her contribution that remains unchanged from the first edition of this textbook.

Table 9-1. National Cancer Institute Domains of Complementary and Alternative Therapies

Domains of CAM	Definition	Examples
Alternative medical systems	Systems built upon completed systems of theory and practice	Traditional Chinese medicine (acupuncture), homeopathy, naturopathy
Manipulative and body-based methods	Methods based on manipulation and/or movement of one or more parts of the body	Chiropractic, therapeutic massage, reflexology
Energy therapies	Therapies involving the use of energy fields	Reiki, therapeutic touch, magnet therapy
Mind-body interventions	Techniques designed to enhance the mind's capacity to affect bodily function and symptoms	Meditation, hypnosis, art therapy, imagery, relaxation therapy, support groups, music therapy, cognitive-behavioral therapy, prayer, dance therapy, psychoneuroimmunology, aromatherapy
Movement therapy	Modalities used to improve patterns of bodily movement	T'ai Chi, Feldenkrais, Alexander technique, QiGong, Trager method, applied kinesiology
Nutritional therapeutics	Assortment of nutrients and non-nutrient and bioactive food components that are used as chemopreventive agents, and the use of specific foods or diets as cancer prevention or treatment strategies	Dietary regimens such as macrobiotics, vegetarianism, Gerson therapy, Kelley/Gonzalez regimen, vitamins, dietary macronutrients, supplements, antioxidants, selenium, coenzyme Q10
Pharmacologic and biologic treatments	Drugs, complex natural products, vaccines, and other biologic interventions not yet accepted in mainstream medicine, as well as off-label use of prescription drugs	Antineoplastons, 714-X, immunoaugmentative therapy, laetrile, hydrazine sulfate, Newcastle disease virus, ozone therapy, enzyme therapy, high doses of vitamin C

(Continued on next page)

Table 9-1. National Cancer Institute Domains of Complementary and Alternative Therapies *(Continued)*		
Domains of CAM	**Definition**	**Examples**
Complex natural products	Subcategory of pharma-cologic and biologic treat-ments consisting of an as-sortment of plant samples (botanicals), extracts of crude natural substances, others	Herbs and herbal extracts, mix-tures of tea polyphenols, shark cartilage, Essiac tea, cordyceps, Sun's Soup, MGN-3

CAM—complementary and alternative medicine

Note. From "Complementary and Alternative Medicine (CAM) Therapies" (pp. 593–594), by C.H. Yarbro, M.H. Frogge, and M. Goodman (Eds.), *Cancer Nursing: Principles and Practice* (6th ed.), 2005, Sudbury, MA: Jones and Bartlett. Copyright 2005 by Jones and Bartlett. Adapted with permission.

Specific Issues Related to Palliative Care

National surveys have confirmed a persisting interest in and use of CAM therapies in the United States and Europe (Eisenberg et al., 1993, 1998). The Office of Alternative Medicine was established in 1992 in response to the continued use of and issues surrounding CAM therapies. This department became the NCCAM in 1998. The NCCAM does not provide referrals to CAM practitioners (NCCAM, 2004).

The White House Commission on Complementary and Alternative Medicine Policy (2002) was established in March 2000 to address issues related to access to and delivery of CAM, priorities for research, and the need for consumer and healthcare provider (HCP) education. In 2003–2004, the Institute of Medicine (IOM) of the National Academies sponsored seven committee meetings to explore scientific, policy, and practice questions that arise from the increasing use of CAM by the American public (IOM, 2004).

Strategies to Promote Use in Palliative Care

Recommending CAM therapies remains challenging for HCPs. Research confirms that HCPs do not offer CAM therapies, and patients do not request them for a variety of reasons, including fear of being dismissed by their HCP and fear of disapproval of family and friends. These and other reasons for withholding information are discussed by Eisenberg (1997) and Decker (2005), who offer algorithms for advising patients regarding CAM therapies (see Figure 9-1).

A Model for Advising Patients and Families

More often, HCPs have patients who request information regarding CAM therapies for a variety of reasons, including symptoms associated with palliative care. A

Figure 9-1. Discussing Complementary and Alternative Medicine Therapies With Patients

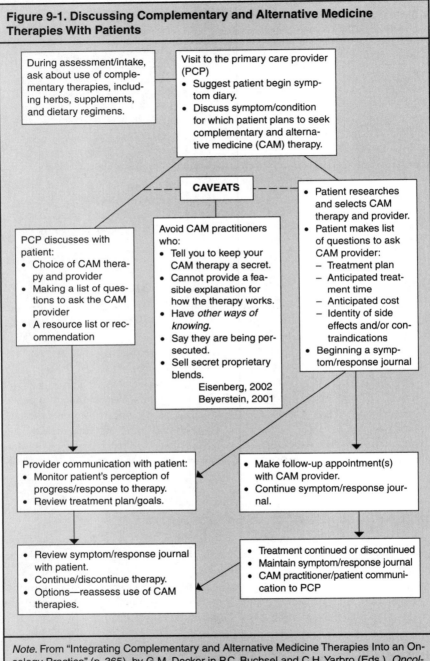

During assessment/intake, ask about use of complementary therapies, including herbs, supplements, and dietary regimens.

Visit to the primary care provider (PCP)
- Suggest patient begin symptom diary.
- Discuss symptom/condition for which patient plans to seek complementary and alternative medicine (CAM) therapy.

CAVEATS

PCP discusses with patient:
- Choice of CAM therapy and provider
- Making a list of questions to ask the CAM provider
- A resource list or recommendation

Avoid CAM practitioners who:
- Tell you to keep your CAM therapy a secret.
- Cannot provide a feasible explanation for how the therapy works.
- Have *other ways of knowing.*
- Say they are being persecuted.
- Sell secret proprietary blends.
  Eisenberg, 2002
  Beyerstein, 2001

- Patient researches and selects CAM therapy and provider.
- Patient makes list of questions to ask CAM provider:
  – Treatment plan
  – Anticipated treatment time
  – Anticipated cost
  – Identity of side effects and/or contraindications
- Beginning a symptom/response journal

Provider communication with patient:
- Monitor patient's perception of progress/response to therapy.
- Review treatment plan/goals.

- Make follow-up appointment(s) with CAM provider.
- Continue symptom/response journal.

- Review symptom/response journal with patient.
- Continue/discontinue therapy.
- Options—reassess use of CAM therapies.

- Treatment continued or discontinued
- Maintain symptom/response journal
- CAM practitioner/patient communication to PCP

common difficulty is that patients and families tend to equate "natural" with "safe" and frequently have misconceptions regarding a particular therapy or category of therapies before they have any discussion with their HCP. The safe and appropriate use of a CAM therapy is as important in palliative care as during any other time in the continuum of care. Because of the widespread availability and affordability of many CAM therapies, increased integration of these therapies into palliative care is inevitable. Selected sponsored Web sites, peer-reviewed journals indexed in MEDLINE®, and databases are listed in Table 9-2.

A legal definition of *complementary and alternative medicine* that is inclusive and official does not exist. The issue of liability when a licensed practitioner refers a patient to a CAM provider who is not licensed is of concern. Regulatory arenas will address informed consent, licensure versus certification or registration, scopes of practice, malpractice, and professional discipline.

Examples of Integrative Therapies Used in Palliative Care

A. Pain (Ahmed, Craig, White, & Huber, 1998; Dalton, Keefe, Carlson, & Youngblood, 2004; Kwekkeboom, 2003; Moyer, 2004; Natural Standard, 2007; Physician's Desk Reference, 2002; Terkelsen, Anderson, Molgaard, Hansen, & Jensen, 2004)
  1. **Level I—high level of evidence**
     a) Acupuncture
     b) Cognitive-behavioral treatment
     c) Massage
     d) Music and distraction—procedural pain
  2. **Level II—moderate level of evidence**
     a) Chiropractic (except cervical manipulation)
     b) Relaxation with guided imagery (Avoid in patients with a history of physical or sexual abuse, post-traumatic stress disorder [PTSD], clinical depression, or bipolar disorder.)
     c) Topical capsaicin

B. Anorexia (Loprinzi, Goldberg, et al., 1994; Loprinzi, Kuross, et al., 1994; Natural Medicine Comprensive Database, 2007; Natural Standard, 2007; Physician's Desk Reference, 2001; Wigmore et al., 1996)
  1. **Level I—high level of evidence**
     a) Proven to be effective
        (1) Eicosapentanoic acid
        (2) Soy
     b) Proven to be ineffective
        (1) Hydrazine sulfate
        (2) Herbals: Alfalfa, astragalus, betel nut, black cohosh, blessed thistle, chamomile, cranberry, dandelion, devil's claw, Essiac, eyebright, fenugreek, ginseng, hawthorn, hops, kava, lavender, oleander, peppermint, sorrel, thyme, turmeric, valerian, white horehound

Table 9-2. Sources of Reliable Cancer Complementary and Alternative Medicine Information—Select Sites

Source	Web Site
Organizations	
American Cancer Society	www.cancer.org
American Society of Clinical Oncology	www.asco.org
Cancer Information Service	http://cis.nci.nih.gov
Cancer Patient Education Network	www.cancerpatienteducation.org
Dana-Farber Cancer Institute Zakim Center for Integrated Therapies	www.dana-farber.org/pat/support/zakim_default.asp
Johns Hopkins Center for Complementary and Alternative Medicine	www.hopkinsmedicine.org/CAM/links.html
MedlinePlus	http://medlineplus.gov
National Center for Complementary and Alternative Medicine	http://nccam.nih.gov
National Institutes of Health	www.nih.gov
Office of Cancer Complementary and Alternative Medicine	www3.cancer.gov/occam
Office of Dietary Supplements	http://ods.od.nih.gov
People Living with Cancer	www.plwc.org
Rosenthal Center for Complementary and Alternative Medicine	http://rosenthal.hs.columbia.edu
U.S. Food and Drug Administration	www.fda.gov
Journals	
Alternative & Complementary Therapies	www.liebertpub.com/publication.aspx?pub_id=3
British Medical Journal	www.bmj.com
Clinical Journal of Oncology Nursing	www.ons.org/publications/journals/CJON
Integrative Cancer Therapies	www.sagepub.com/journal.aspx?pid=286
Journal of Alternative and Complementary Medicine	www.liebertpub.com/publication.aspx?pub_id=26
Journal of Clinical Oncology	www.jco.org

(Continued on next page)

Table 9-2. Sources of Reliable Cancer Complementary and Alternative Medicine Information—Select Sites *(Continued)*	
Source	**Web Site**
JAMA	http://jama.ama-assn.org
Oncology Nursing Forum	www.ons.org/publications/journals/ONF
Seminars in Oncology Nursing	www.seminarsinoncologynursing.com
Databases	
American Botanical Council	www.herbalgram.org
ClinicalTrials.gov	http://clinicaltrials.gov/ct
International Bibliographic Information on Dietary Supplements	http://ods.od.nih.gov/Health_Information/IBIDS.aspx
Micromedex	www.micromedex.com/products/hcs
Natural Medicines Comprehensive Database	www.naturaldatabase.com
Natural Standard	www.naturalstandard.com
PDQ® (Physician Data Query, National Cancer Institute)	http://cancer.gov/cancerinfo/pdq
The Cochrane Collaboration	www.cochrane.org
U.S. Food and Drug Administration	www.fda.gov

    2. **Level II—moderate level of evidence**
      (conflicting)
      a) Bromelian
      b) Omega-3 fatty acids, fish oil, alpha-linolenic acid
    3. **Level III—low level of evidence**
      Spirulina

C. Depression (Cassileth & Vickers, 2003; Crevenna et al., 2003; Ernst, 2001; Fellowes, Barnes, & Wilkinson, 2004; Hadfield, 2001; Jorm, Christensen, Griffiths, & Rodgers, 2002; Kasper & Dienel, 2002; Krampen, Main, & Waelbroeck, 1991; Kwekkeboom, 2003; Moyer, Rounds, & Hannum, 2004; Natural Standard, 2007; Roschke et al., 2000; Zappa & Cassileth, 2003)
    1. **Level I—high level of evidence**
      a) Acupuncture
      b) Herbal therapies
      c) St. John's wort is effective in the treatment of mild to moderate depression; not effective for severe depression

    d) Autogenic training as a complementary therapy
    e) Music therapy
    f) Massage (This therapy should be used with caution in patients with a history of sexual or physical abuse, PTSD, or other psychiatric disorders.)
    g) Aerobic exercise
2. **Level II—moderate level of evidence**
    a) Aromatherapy as complementary to antidepressants and massage
    b) Relaxation

Patient Outcomes

A. Patient has improved sense of well-being, such as
   1. Absence of or decreased pain
   2. Improvement in mood
   3. Improved sleep, relaxation, and relationship with peers and family.

B. Patient experiences realization or perception of possible anticancer effects of a particular CAM therapy, such as a decrease in symptom(s).

C. Patient verbalizes a sense of improved quality or quantity of life, such as
   1. Improved sleep.
   2. Increased activities of daily living.

D. Patient verbalizes improved sense of control: Evidence of decision making is present.

E. Patient verbalizes improved peer or family relationships: Improvement or increase in communication occurs with peers and/or family.

References

Ahmed, H.E., Craig, W.F., White, P.F., & Huber, P. (1998). Percutaneous electrical nerve stimulation (PENS): A complementary therapy for the management of pain secondary to bony metastasis. *Clinical Journal of Pain, 14,* 320–323.

Cassileth, B.R., & Vickers, A.J. (2003). Complementary and alternative therapies. *Urologic Clinics of North America, 30,* 369–376.

Crevenna, R., Zielinski, C., Keilani, M.Y., Schmidinger, M., Bittner, C., Nuhr, M., et al. (2003). [Aerobic endurance training for cancer patients]. *Wiener Medizinische Wochenschrift, 153,* 212–216.

Dalton, J.A., Keefe, F.J., Carlson, J., & Youngblood, R. (2004). Tailoring cognitive-behavioral treatment for cancer pain. *Pain Management Nursing, 5,* 3–18.

Decker, G. (2005). Integrating complementary and alternative medicine therapies into an oncology practice. In P.C. Buchsel (Ed.), *Oncology nursing in the ambulatory setting: Issues and models of care* (pp. 355–375). Sudbury, MA: Jones and Bartlett.

Eisenberg, D.M. (1997). Advising patients who seek alternative medical therapies. *Annals of Internal Medicine, 127,* 61–69.

Eisenberg, D.M., Davis, R.B., Ettner, S.L., Appel, S., Wilkey, S., Van Rompay, M., et al. (1998). Trends in alternative medicine use in the United States, 1990–1997: Results of a follow-up national survey. *JAMA, 280,* 1569–1575.

Eisenberg, D.M., Kessler, R.C., Foster, C., Norlock, F.E., Calkins, D.R., & Delbanco, T.L. (1993). Unconventional medicine in the United States. Prevalence, costs, and patterns of use. *New England Journal of Medicine, 328,* 246–252.

Ernst, E. (Ed.). (2001). *The desktop guide to complementary and alternative medicine: An evidence-based approach.* Edinburgh, Scotland: Mosby.

Fellowes, D., Barnes, K., & Wilkinson, S. (2004). Aromatherapy and massage for symptom relief in patients with cancer. *Cochrane Database of Systematic Reviews 2004,* Issue 3. Article No: CD002287. DOI: 10.1002/14651858.CD002287.pub2.

Hadfield, N. (2001). The role of aromatherapy massage in reducing anxiety in patients with malignant brain tumours. *International Journal of Palliative Nursing, 7,* 279–285.

Institute of Medicine of the National Academies. (2004). *Use of complementary and alternative medicine (CAM) by the American public.* Retrieved May 16, 2007, from http://www.iom.edu/ CMS/3793/4829/24431.aspx

Jorm, A.F., Christensen, H., Griffiths, K.M., & Rodgers, B. (2002). Effectiveness of complementary and self-help treatments for depression. *Medical Journal of Australia, 176*(Suppl.), 84–96.

Kasper, S., & Dienel, A. (2002). Cluster analysis of symptoms during antidepressant treatment with Hypericum extract in mildly to moderately depressed out-patients. A meta-analysis of data from three randomized, placebo-controlled trials. *Psychopharmacology (Berl.), 164,* 301–308.

Krampen, G., Main, C., & Waelbroeck, O. (1991). [Optimizing the learning process in short-term autogenic training by practice protocols]. *Zeitschrift für klinische Psychologie, Psychopathologie und Psychotherapie, 39,* 33–45.

Kwekkeboom, K.L. (2003). Music versus distraction for procedural pain and anxiety in patients with cancer. *Oncology Nursing Forum, 30,* 433–440.

Loprinzi, C.L., Goldberg, R.M., Su, J.Q., Mailliard, J.A., Kuross, S.A., Maksymiuk, A.W., et al. (1994). Placebo-controlled trial of hydrazine sulfate in patients with newly diagnosed non-small-cell lung cancer. *Journal of Clinical Oncology, 12,* 1126–1129.

Loprinzi, C.L., Kuross, S.A., O'Fallon, J.R., Gesme, D.H., Jr., Gerstner, J.B., Rospond, R.M., et al. (1994). Randomized placebo-controlled evaluation of hydrazine sulfate in patients with advanced colorectal cancer. *Journal of Clinical Oncology, 12,* 1121–1125.

Moyer, C.A., Rounds, J., & Hannum, J.W. (2004). A meta-analysis of massage therapy research. *Psychological Bulletin, 130,* 3–18.

National Cancer Institute. (2004a). *Levels of evidence for human studies of cancer complementary and alternative medicine.* Retrieved May 18, 2007, from http://www.nci.nih.gov/cancerinfo/pdq/ levels-evidence-cam

National Cancer Institute. (2004b). *NCI cancer facts: How to evaluate health information on the Internet.* Retrieved May 18, 2007, from http://cis.nci.nih.gov/fact/2_10.html

National Center for Complementary and Alternative Medicine. (2004). *National Center for Complementary and Alternative Medicine.* Retrieved May 18, 2007, from http://nccam.nih.gov/

Natural Medicine Comprehensive Database. (2007). *Natural medicine comprehensive database.* Retrieved May 18, 2007, from http://www.naturaldatabase.com

Natural Standard. (2007). *Natural standard database: Foods, herbs, and supplements.* Retrieved May 18, 2007, from http://www.naturalstandard.com

Oncology Nursing Society. (2006). *Position on the use of complementary, alternative, and integrative therapies in cancer care.* Retrieved May 18, 2007, from http://www.ons.org/publications/positions/ documents/pdfs/AlternativeTherapies.pdf

Physician's Desk Reference. (2001). *PDR for nutritional supplements.* Montvale, NJ: Medical Economics Co.

Physician's Desk Reference. (2002). *PDR for herbal medicines* (2nd ed.). Montvale, NJ: Medical Economics Co.

Roschke, J., Wolf, C., Muller, M.J., Wagner, P., Mann, K., Grozinger, M., et al. (2000). The benefit from whole body acupuncture in major depression. *Journal of Affective Disorders, 57,* 73–81.

Terkelsen, A.J., Andersen, O.K., Molgaard, H., Hansen, J., & Jensen, T.S. (2004). Mental stress inhibits pain perception and heart rate variability but not a nociceptive withdrawal reflex. *Acta Physiologica Scandinavica, 180,* 405–414.

White House Commission on Complementary and Alternative Medicine Policy. (2002, March). *White House Commission on Complementary and Alternative Medicine Policy final report.* Retrieved May 18, 2007, from http://whccamp.hhs.gov/sfc.html

Wigmore, S.J., Ross, J.A., Falconer, J.S., Plester, C.E., Tisdale, M.J., Carter, D.C., et al. (1996). The effect of polyunsaturated fatty acids on the progress of cachexia in patients with pancreatic cancer. *Nutrition, 12*(Suppl. 1), 27–30.

Zappa, S.B., & Cassileth, B.R. (2003). Complementary approaches to palliative oncological care. *Journal of Nursing Care Quality, 18,* 22–26.

Constipation

Pamela Spencer, BA, MSN, BSN, FNP

Definition

Constipation is a condition that features abnormal bowel movements, which may include straining, hard stools, decreased frequency, and a feeling of incomplete evacuation. The frequency of "normal" bowel movements ranges from 3–12 per week; two or fewer bowel movements per week is considered abnormal (Kearney, 2003). Constipation is the most prevalent digestive complaint in the United States and is a frequent problem in patients with progressive illness in the palliative care setting. It occurs in as many as two-thirds of palliative care patients (Lenz, 2003). Chronic constipation may lead to rectal prolapse, hemorrhoidal bleeding, or development of an anal fissure. Fecal impaction may produce colonic obstruction or stercoral ulcers, which can bleed and perforate (Summers, 2005).

Pathophysiology and Etiology

The etiology of constipation is multifactorial, given the complexity of colonic function and the defecatory process. Constipation can occur as a result of abnormal motor function of the large intestine, which may be caused by systemic disease, medications, or primary motor disorders of the bowel. Alternatively, abnormalities of the muscular structures of the anorectum (pelvic floor dysfunction) may lead to abnormal defecation and constipation (Kearney, 2003). Other contributing factors to constipation include immobility, dietary changes, chemical imbalances, ascites, adhesions, or psychological concerns, including stress, anxiety, and embarrassment (Bennett & Cresswell, 2003; Heidrich, 2007). Perhaps the most common cause of constipation in the palliative care setting is drug therapy, with opioids being the usual etiology (Lenz, 2003).

Manifestations

- Rectal bleeding
- Nausea

The author would like to acknowledge Kimberly A. Zielke, MD, for her contributions that remain unchanged from the first edition of this textbook.

- Anal pain
- Malaise
- Abdominal bloating
- Headache
- Abdominal pain and distention
- Hemorrhoids
- Ascites
- Dry, hard stool
- Confusion
- Straining to move bowels
- Flatulence

(Heidrich, 2007; Yamada et al., 2005)

Management

A. Death is not imminent. (Brandt, Schoenfeld, & Prather, 2005; Klaschik, Nauck, & Ostgathe, 2003; Lussier & Portenoy, 2004; Sykes, 2003; Yamada et al., 2005)
  1. **Level I—high level of evidence**
     a) Several prophylactic measures should be employed when possible, including maintaining general symptom control, encouraging activity, maintaining adequate oral intake, anticipating the constipating effects of drugs (altering treatment or starting a laxative prophylactically), and creating a favorable environment (e.g., providing privacy, positioning the patient upright).
     b) The choice of laxative depends on the characteristics of the patient's stool and the individual's response to therapy. Hard, dry stool requires more softener. Stool that is difficult to pass requires more stimulant; a patient experiencing abdominal cramping may require less stimulant.
        (1) Casanthrol and docusate sodium (Peri-Colace®) ($)—1–2 tablets po bid; no ceiling effect; also available in syrup
        (2) Senna (Senokot®) ($)—1–3 tablets po two or four times a day, may titrate both senna and docusate sodium until bowel movement occurs
        (3) Senna concentrate and docusate sodium (Senokot S®) ($$)—same as dosing above for senna.
     c) When the amount of combination stimulant and softener medications produces distressing side effects (e.g., cramping), an osmotic agent should be added, such as the following (starting dose for all: 15 ml po bid).
        (1) Milk of magnesia ($)
        (2) Sorbitol ($)
        (3) Lactulose (Chronulac®) ($$)
        (4) Polyethylene glycol (Miralax®) ($$)—Use 1 heaping tablespoon (17 g) in 8 oz. of fluid daily.

    d) Suppositories (glycerin, bisacodyl) or enemas (saline, oil retention, milk and molasses) ($)—can be considered when the patient requires assistance with evacuation. Suppositories may be adequate if only moderate softening is required. In patients whose rectal vault is loaded with soft stool, a suppository may assist in initial defecation, thus relieving some rectal discomfort.

    e) When the offending medication is required for symptom control, a change to a medication with the potential for fewer side effects should be considered.

  2. **Level II—moderate level of evidence**
(Lenz, 2003; Yamada et al., 2005)

    a) Nonpharmacologic treatment in some cases includes biofeedback techniques.

    b) Empty distended rectum.

B. Death is imminent.

  Level I—high level of evidence
(Lenz, 2003; McMillan, 2002)

  1. Even when a patient has had minimal intake for days or weeks, the bowels still need to move to provide comfort. Stool is not only a formation of food but also includes metabolic wastes. A patient who is dying may experience dysphagia, so a suppository or enema may be more useful than oral medication.

  2. If the patient is experiencing increased confusion, abdominal bloating, cramping, or pain, the following interventions should be considered. Keeping the rectal vault clear of stool is important when the rectum is needed for medication administration and bioavailability.

    a) Bisacodyl suppository (Dulcolax®) ($)

    b) Saline enema (Fleet®) ($)

Patient Outcomes

A. Medications that cause constipation are recognized and adjusted.

B. A prophylactic bowel regimen is prescribed when prescribing opioids.

C. Symptoms of agitation, confusion, restlessness, abdominal bloating, nausea, and pain are recognized as indicators of constipation.

References

Bennett, M., & Creswell, H. (2003). Factors influencing constipation in advanced cancer patients: A prospective study of opioid dose, Dantron dose and physical functioning. *Palliative Medicine, 17,* 418–422.

Brandt, L., Schoenfeld, P., & Prather, C. (2005). Evidence-based position statement on the management of chronic constipation in North America. *American Journal of Gastroenterology, 100*(Suppl. 1), S1–S11.

Heidrich, D.E. (2007). Constipation. In K.K. Kuebler, D.E. Heidrich, & P. Esper (Eds.), *Palliative and end-of-life-care: Clinical practice guidelines* (2nd. ed., pp. 287–300). St. Louis, MO: Elsevier Saunders.

Kearney, D. (2003). Approach to the patient with gastrointestinal disorders. In S. Friedman, K. McQuaid, & J. Grendell (Eds.), *Current diagnosis and treatment in gastroenterology* (2nd ed., pp. 1–33). New York: McGraw-Hill.

Klaschik, E., Nauck, F., & Ostgathe, C. (2003). Constipation: Modern laxative therapy. *Supportive Care in Cancer, 11,* 679–685.

Lenz, K.L. (2003). The pharmacology of symptom control. In G. Taylor & J. Kurent (Eds.), *A clinician's guide to palliative care* (2nd ed., pp. 19–46). Malden, MA: Blackwell Science.

Lussier, D., & Portenoy, R.K. (2004). Adjuvant analgesics in pain management. In D. Doyle, G. Hanks, N.I. Cherny, & K. Calman (Eds.), *Oxford textbook of palliative medicine* (3rd ed., pp. 349–378). New York: Oxford University Press.

McMillan, S.C. (2002). Presence and severity of constipation in hospice patients with advanced cancer. *American Journal of Hospice and Palliative Care, 19,* 426–430.

Summers, R.W. (2005). Approach to the patient with constipation. In T. Yamada, W. Hasler, J. Inadomi, M. Anderson, & R. Brown (Eds.), *Handbook of gastroenterology* (2nd ed., pp. 87–94). Philadelphia: Lippincott Williams & Wilkins.

Sykes, N.P. (2003). Constipation and diarrhea. In D. Doyle, G. Hanks, & N. Cherny (Eds.), *Oxford textbook of palliative medicine* (3rd ed., pp. 483–496). New York: Oxford University Press.

Cough

Jennifer Fournier, RN, MSN, AOCN®, CHPN

Definition

Cough is an explosive expulsion of inspired air that clears the airway with a velocity that can be as great as 500 miles per hour (Irwin, Ownbey, Cagle, Baker, & Fraire, 2006; McCool, 2006). Generally, coughing is a protective mechanism for the lungs and bronchial tree but also can be the result of certain disorders (Fournier, 2007; Keenleyside & Vora, 2006). The established categorization of cough is based on duration: acute cough (< 3 weeks), subacute cough (3–8 weeks), and chronic cough (> 8 weeks) (Fournier; Pratter & Abouzgheib, 2006).

Pathophysiology and Etiology

Vagal afferent nerves govern the involuntary cough reflex. Cough also may be controlled voluntarily via the cortex (Bolser, 2006; Fitzgerald, 2007; Fournier, 2007; Irwin, Baumann, et al., 2006; Keenleyside & Vora, 2006). Effective cough relies more on strong expiratory musculature than strong inspiratory musculature. Ineffective cough may result in pneumonia, atelectasis, or respiratory failure (McCool, 2006).

Cough is one of the most prevalent symptoms in the last year of life (Doorenbos, Given, Given, & Verbitsky, 2006; Keenleyside & Vora, 2006; McMillan, Dunbar, & Zhang, 2007) and is the most common symptom for which medical care is sought (Irwin, 2006; Pratter & Abouzgheib, 2006). Frequently, more than a single cause of cough exists (Pratter, Brightling, Boulet, & Irwin, 2006). A worsening cough in the palliative care patient may signal progression of disease. The palliative care patient may experience sleep disturbances that can be attributed to cough (Vena et al., 2006). Also, cough can lead to difficulty in eating, conversing, and socializing and an overall decreased quality of life.

Life-threatening conditions such as congestive heart failure, cardiac tamponade, superior vena cava syndrome, pneumonia, and pulmonary embolism may present with cough as a symptom in the palliative care patient (Fournier, 2007; Pratter et al., 2006). Non–life-threatening etiologies of cough include upper airway cough

The author would like to acknowledge Beth Cohen, RNC, ARNP, MSN, for her contribution that remains unchanged from the first edition of this textbook.

syndrome (UACS), asthma, gastroesophageal reflux disease (GERD), angiotensin-converting enzyme inhibitors (ACEIs), bronchitis, bronchiectasis, common cold, chronic obstructive pulmonary disease (COPD), viral or bacterial upper or lower airway infections, lung tumors, and environmental irritants (Chang, Lasserson, Gaffney, Connor, & Garske, 2006; Fournier; Irwin, Ownbey, et al., 2006; McCrory & Lewis, 2006; Panpanich, Lerttrakamnon, & Laopaiboon, 2004; Schroeder & Fahey, 2004).

Noninfectious subacute cough should be managed as a chronic cough (Irwin, Baumann, et al., 2006). Chronic cough may be caused by airway mast cell activation and possibly thought of as the result of an airway itch that may be brought on by the act of coughing itself (Gibson, 2004; Irwin, Ownbey, et al., 2006). The use of an ACEI can induce chronic cough in up to 35% of patients (Dicpinigaitis, 2006; Irwin, Ownbey, et al.). By far, the most likely causes of chronic cough in nonsmoking patients with a normal chest x-ray and who are not taking an ACEI are UACS, GERD, or asthma either individually or together (Pratter, 2006b). Of these, the most common cause of chronic cough is UACS, previously called postnasal drip syndrome (Pratter & Abouzgheib, 2006). UACS frequently is the result of the common cold and can be traced to one of at least 200 viruses that infect adults at the rate of two to four colds per year (Pratter, 2006a). GERD can be the source of chronic cough in 41% of patients presenting with cough as a complaint (Chang et al., 2006). Cough related to asthma may be found in 16% of patients with chronic cough (Pratter & Abouzgheib).

A detailed history and thorough physical examination are vital to determine the cause of cough. The history will show comorbidities, tobacco use, aggravating and alleviating factors, and most importantly, the effect on the palliative care patient's quality of life. Significant assessments include the duration and quality of the cough, sputum production and character, and the condition of the airway (Fournier, 2007; Keenleyside & Vora, 2006). When the common causes of cough have been exhausted, it may be prudent to consider the possibility of a foreign body in the airway, environmental irritants, or drug-induced cough (Irwin, Baumann, et al., 2006; Tarlo, 2006).

Manifestations

- Increased blood pressure
- Sleep disturbances
- Sore throat
- Hemoptysis
- Abdominal and chest pain
- Weakness
- Tiredness
- Anxiety
- Rib fractures
- Impaired socialization
- Syncope

- Vomiting
- Urinary incontinence

(Fournier, 2007; Irwin, Ownbey, et al., 2006; Keenleyside & Vora, 2006)

Management

A. Death is not imminent.
   1. **Level I—high level of evidence**
      (Ducharme & Di Salvio, 2003; Fahey, Smucny, Becker, & Glazier, 2004; Fournier, 2007; Hospice Pharmacia, 2006; Irwin, Baumann, et al., 2006; Keenleyside & Vora, 2006; Lester, Macbeth, Toy, & Coles, 2006; Olin, 2008; Panpanich et al., 2004; Pratter & Abouzgheib, 2006; Pratter et al., 2006; Smucny, Becker, & Glazier, 2006; *Tarascon Pocket Pharmacopoeia,* 2004)
      a) Cough related to UACS (formerly known as postnasal drip)
         (1) Antihistamine and decongestant
            (a) Chlorpheniramine ($) or brompheniramine ($)—4 mg po every four to six hours (maximum 24 mg daily) in combination with pseudoephedrine
            (b) Pseudoephedrine ($)—60 mg po every four to six hours (maximum 240 mg daily)
         (2) Cough suppressants for nonproductive cough (short-term)
            (a) Dextromethorphan ($)—10–30 mg po every four hours (maximum 120 mg daily)
            (b) Codeine ($)—10–20 mg po every four to six hours
            (c) Hydrocodone ($)—5 mg po every six hours
      b) Cough related to lower respiratory tract bacterial infection
         (1) Antibiotics
            (a) Amoxicillin (Amoxil®) ($)—500 mg po three times a day is as effective as azithromycin
            (b) Azithromycin (Zithromax®) ($$)—500 mg po on day one, then 250 mg po daily for four days
         (2) Increase fluids.
      c) Cough related to asthma
         (1) Inhaled corticosteroids and β-agonists
            (a) Beclomethasone (QVAR®) ($$)—one to four puffs bid (max 16 puffs/day) in combination with albuterol
            (b) Albuterol (Proventil®) ($)—two puffs every four to six hours, as needed
         (2) Leukotriene modifiers, for when asthmatic cough is refractory
            (a) Montelukast (Singulair®) ($$$)—10 mg po nightly
            (b) Zafirlukast (Accolate®) ($$)—20 mg po bid at least one hour before or two hours after meals
      d) Cough related to stable bronchitis
         (1) Bronchodilators
            (a) Ipratropium (Atrovent®) ($$)—two puffs four times a day

  (b) Theophylline sustained release ($)—200–300 mg po bid

   i) Monitor therapeutic blood levels.

   ii) Many drug interactions are possible.

 (2) Cough suppressants for short-term use

  (a) Dextromethorphan ($)—10–30 mg po every four hours (max 120 mg/day)

  (b) Codeine ($)—10–20 mg po every four to six hours

e) Acute exacerbation of chronic bronchitis

 (1) Antibiotics—Determining if infection is bacterial or viral is difficult; therefore, antibiotics may have a beneficial effect, but the likely side effects and cost should be considered.

  (a) Amoxicillin (Amoxil) ($)—500 mg po three times a day is as effective as

  (b) Azithromycin (Zithromax) ($$)—500 mg po on day one, then 250 mg po daily for four days

  (c) Erythromycin (E-mycin®) ($)—500 mg po four times a day for 10 days

  (d) Doxycycline (Vibramycin®) ($)—100 mg po bid for 10 days

  (e) Levofloxacin (Levaquin®) ($$$)—750 mg po daily for five days

 (2) β-agonist bronchodilator

  (a) Albuterol (Proventil) ($)—two puffs every four to six hours, as needed

  (b) Use is controversial in patients without asthma.

 (3) Anticholinergic bronchodilator: Ipratropium (Atrovent) ($$)—two puffs four times a day

 (4) Cough suppressants for short-term use

  (a) Dextromethorphan ($)—10–30 mg po every four hours (max 120 mg/day)

  (b) Codeine ($)—10–20 mg po every four to six hours

 (5) Short course of oral corticosteroids

  (a) Dexamethasone ($)—4–8 mg po daily

  (b) Prednisone ($)—20–60 mg po daily; taper to lowest effective dose.

f) Cough related to subacute (three to eight weeks duration) postinfectious cough

 (1) Anticholinergic bronchodilator: Ipratropium (Atrovent) ($$)—two to three puffs four times daily

 (2) Inhaled corticosteroids, if failed ipratropium

  (a) Beclomethasone (QVAR) ($$)—one to four puffs bid (maximum 16 puffs daily)

  (b) Flunisolide (AeroBid®) ($$)—two to four puff bid (maximum eight puffs daily)

 (3) Short-term oral corticosteroids for severe cough

  (a) Dexamethasone ($)—4–8 mg po daily

    (b) Prednisone ($)—20–60 mg po daily; taper to lowest effective dose.

  (4) Cough suppressants

    (a) Dextromethorphan ($)—10–30 mg po every four hours (max 120 mg/day)

    (b) Codeine ($)—10–20 mg po every four to six hours

 g) Cough related to lung tumors

  (1) External beam radiation ($$$)

  (2) Chemotherapy ($$$)

2. **Level II—moderate level of evidence**

(Chang et al., 2006; Homsi, Walsh, & Nelson, 2001; Hospice Pharmacia, 2006; Irwin, Baumann, et al., 2006; *Tarascon Pocket Pharmacopoeia, 2004*)

 a) Cough related to UACS

  (1) Expectorant: Guaifenesin ($)—5–10 ml po every four hours around the clock or as needed for productive cough

  (2) Suppressant

    (a) Guaifenesin DM ($)—5–10 ml po every four hours around the clock or as needed for nonproductive cough

    (b) Promethazine DM ($)—5–10 ml po every four hours around the clock or as needed for nonproductive cough

 b) Chronic cough related to GERD

  (1) Proton pump inhibitor

    (a) Omeprazole (Prilosec®) ($$$)—20–40 mg po daily

    (b) Lansoprazole (Prevacid®) ($$$)—15–30 mg po daily

  (2) H_2 antagonists

    (a) Famotidine (Pepcid®) ($$)—20–40 mg po bid

    (b) Ranitidine (Zantac®) ($$)—150–300 mg po bid

 c) Cough related to bronchiectasis

  (1) Bronchodilators when airflow obstruction or bronchial hyperactivity present

    (a) Albuterol (Proventil) ($)—two puffs every four to six hours, as needed

    (b) Ipratropium (Atrovent) ($$)—two puffs four times a day

  (2) Chest physiotherapy with ineffective cough and hypersecretion of mucus

 d) Cough related to lung tumors: Cough suppressant

  (1) Hydrocodone ($)—5–10 mg po three to four times daily

  (2) Benzonatate (Tessalon Perles®) ($)—Non-narcotic 100–200 mg po three times a day

3. **Level III—low level of evidence**

(Beers & Jones, 2006; Irwin, Baumann, et al., 2006; McCool & Rosen, 2006)

 a) To improve cough in patients with expiratory neuromuscular weakness

        (1) Manually assisted cough (only with no accompanying COPD)
        (2) Expiratory muscle training
     b) Huffing for patients with COPD or cystic fibrosis
     c) Chest percussion for frail, older adult patients with pneumonia

B. Death is imminent. (National Comprehensive Cancer Network, 2006)
   1. Discontinue unnecessary treatments.
   2. Provide symptom management and comfort measures.
   3. Ensure privacy and time with family.
   4. Educate the patient and family regarding the dying process.
   5. Provide psychosocial support.

Patient Outcomes

A. Cough is alleviated.

B. Breathing is effective.

C. Open airways are maintained.

D. Comfort is sustained.

References

Beers, M.H., & Jones, T.V. (Eds.). (2006). Pulmonary infections. In *Merck manual of geriatrics* (3rd ed.). Retrieved May 24, 2007, from http://www.merck.com/mrkshared/mmg/sec10/ch76/ch76a.jsp

Bolser, D.C. (2006). Cough suppressant and pharmacologic protussive therapy: ACCP evidence-based clinical practice guidelines. *Chest, 129*(Suppl. 1), 238S–249S.

Chang, A.B., Lasserson, T.J., Gaffney, J., Connor, F.L., & Garske, L.A. (2006). Gastro-oesophageal reflux treatment for prolonged non-specific cough in children and adults. *Cochrane Database of Systematic Reviews 2005,* Issue 2. Art. No.: CD004823. DOI: 10.1002/14651858. CD004823.pub3.

Dicpinigaitis, P.V. (2006). Angiotensin-converting enzyme inhibitor-induced cough: ACCP evidence-based clinical practice guidelines. *Chest, 129*(Suppl. 1), 169S–173S.

Doorenbos, A.Z., Given, C.W., Given, B., & Verbitsky, N. (2006). Symptom experience in the last year of life among individuals with cancer. *Journal of Pain and Symptom Management, 32,* 403–412.

Ducharme, F.M., & DiSalvio, F. (2003, October). Anti-leukotriene agents compared to inhaled corticosteroids in the management of recurrent and/or chronic asthma in adults and children. *Cochrane Database of Systematic Reviews 2000,* Issue 3. Art. No.: CD002314. DOI: 10.1002/14651858. CD002314.pub2.

Fahey, T., Smucny, J., Becker, L., & Glazier, R. (2004, August). Antibiotics for acute bronchitis. *Cochrane Database of Systematic Reviews 1997,* Issue 4. Art. No.: CD000245. DOI: 10.1002/14651858. CD000245.pub2.

Fitzgerald, M. (2007, January). Diagnosing and managing cough. *American Nurse Today, 2,* 44.

Fournier, J. (2007). Cough. In K.K. Kuebler, D.E. Heidrich, & P. Esper (Eds.), *Palliative and end-of-life care: Clinical practice guidelines* (2nd ed., pp. 301–313). St. Louis, MO: Elsevier Saunders.

Gibson, P.G. (2004). Cough is an airway itch? *American Journal of Respiratory and Critical Care Medicine, 169,* 1–2.

Homsi, J., Walsh, D., & Nelson, K.A. (2001). Important drugs for cough in advanced cancer. *Supportive Care in Cancer, 9,* 565–574.

Hospice Pharmacia. (2006). *Medication use guidelines* (8th ed.). Philadelphia: Author.

Irwin, R.S. (2006). Introduction to the diagnosis and management of cough: ACCP evidence-based clinical practice guidelines. *Chest, 129*(Suppl. 1), 25S–27S.

Irwin, R.S., Baumann, M.H., Bolser, D.C., Boulet, L., Braman, S.S., Brightling, C.E., et al. (2006). Diagnosis and management of cough executive summary: ACCP evidence-based clinical practice guidelines. *Chest, 129*(Suppl. 1) 1S–23S.

Irwin, R.S., Ownbey, R., Cagle, P.T., Baker, S., & Fraire, A.E. (2006). Interpreting the histopathology of chronic cough: ACCP evidence-based clinical practice guidelines. *Chest, 129*(Suppl. 1), 362S–370S.

Keenleyside, G., & Vora, V. (2006). Cough. *Indian Journal of Palliative Care, 12,* 51–55.

Lester, J.F., Macbeth, F.R., Toy, E., & Coles, B. (2006). Palliative radiotherapy regimens for non-small cell lung cancer. *Cochrane Database of Systematic Reviews 2001,* Issue 2. Art. No.: CD002143. DOI: 10.1002/14651858. CD002413.pub2.

McCool, F.D. (2006). Global physiology and pathophysiology of cough: ACCP evidence-based clinical practice guidelines. *Chest, 129*(Suppl. 1), 48S–53S.

McCool, F.D., & Rosen, M.J. (2006). Nonpharmacologic airway clearance therapies: ACCP evidence-based clinical practice guidelines. *Chest, 129*(Suppl. 1), 250S–259S.

McCrory, D.C., & Lewis, S.Z. (2006). Methodology and grading of the evidence for the diagnosis and management of cough: ACCP evidence-based clinical practice guidelines. *Chest, 129*(Suppl. 1), 28S–32S.

McMillan, S.C., Dunbar, S.B., & Zhang, W. (2007). The prevalence of symptoms in hospice patients with end-stage heart disease. *Journal of Hospice and Palliative Nursing, 9,* 124–131.

National Comprehensive Cancer Network. (2006). *NCCN clinical practice guidelines in oncology: Palliative care, version 1.2006.* Retrieved May 22, 2007, from http://www.nccn.org/professionals/physician_gls/PDF/palliative.pdf

Olin, J.L. (2008). Chronic cough. In F.J. Domino (Ed.), *The 5-minute clinical consult 2008* (16th ed., pp. 268–269). Philadelphia: Lippincott Williams & Wilkins.

Panpanich, R., Lerttrakamnon, P., & Laopaiboon, M. (2004). Azithromycin for acute lower respiratory tract infections. *Cochrane Database of Systematic Reviews 2004,* Issue 4. Art. No.: CD001954. DOI: 10.1002/14651858. CD001954.pub3.

Pratter, M.R. (2006a). Cough and the common cold: ACCP evidence-based clinical practice guidelines. *Chest, 129*(Suppl. 1), 72S–74S.

Pratter, M.R. (2006b). Overview of common causes of chronic cough: ACCP evidence-based clinical practice guidelines. *Chest, 129*(Suppl. 1), 59S–62S.

Pratter, M.R., & Abouzgheib, W. (2006). Make the cough go away. *Chest, 129,* 1121–1122.

Pratter, M.R., Brightling, C.E., Boulet, L., & Irwin, R.S. (2006). An empiric integrative approach to the management of cough: ACCP evidence-based clinical practice guidelines. *Chest, 129*(Suppl. 1), 222S–231S.

Schroeder, K., & Fahey, T. (2004, August). Over-the-counter medications for acute cough in children and adults in ambulatory settings. *Cochrane Database of Systematic Reviews 1999,* Issue 1. Art. No.: CD001831. DOI: 10.1002/14651858. CD001831.pub3.

Smucny, J., Becker, L., & Glazier, R. (2006, August). Beta2-agonists for acute bronchitis. *Cochrane Database of Systematic Reviews 2001,* Issue 1. Art. No.: CD001726. DOI: 10.1002/14651858. CD001726.pub3.

Tarascon Pocket Pharmacopoeia (2004 classic shirt-pocket ed.). (2004). Lompoc, CA: Tarascon.

Tarlo, S.M. (2006). Cough: Occupational and environmental considerations: ACCP evidence-based clinical practice guidelines. *Chest, 129*(Suppl. 1), 186S–196S.

Vena, C., Parker, K.P., Allen, R., Bliwise, D.L., Jain, S., & Kimble, L. (2006). Sleep-wake disturbances and quality of life in patients with advanced lung cancer. *Oncology Nursing Forum, 33,* 761–769.

Cultural Competence

Charles E. Kemp, FNP, FAAN

Definitions

Cultural competence is the ability to "perform and obtain positive clinical outcomes in cross-cultural encounters" (Lo & Fung, 2003, p. 162) and includes awareness of one's own culture, recognition of differences between one's own and other cultures, and the ability to "adapt behaviors to appreciate and accommodate those differences" (Drew, 2006, p. 121). Two primary aspects of cultural competence exist.

- *Generic cultural competence* is knowledge and skills applicable to *any* cross-cultural patient or community encounter.
- *Specific cultural competence* is knowledge and skills applicable to patients and communities from specific cultural backgrounds (Flaskerud, 2007; Kemp, 2005).

Both generic and specific cultural competencies include valuing other cultures and are applicable to individual clinicians and institutional policy (Flaskerud, 2007).

Specific Issues Related to Palliative Care

Evidence-based research in cultural competence is focused mainly on intermediate outcomes of short-term interventions, especially in prevention and early detection of cancer and diabetes (Goode, Dunne, & Bronheim, 2006). However, in general, cultural competence on the part of the bedside clinician increases the likelihood of the patient having a "good death" (relatively symptom free and reconciled with self, others, and God or the spiritual), whereas a lack of cultural competence decreases the likelihood of a good death. Likewise, cultural competence on the part of institutions also decreases barriers and disparities and increases the likelihood of a good death (Chrisman, 2007; Kemp & Rasbridge, 2004).

The author would like to acknowledge The Rev. James Deshotels, SJ, APRN, for his contribution that remains unchanged from the first edition of this textbook.

Specific issues related to palliative care and cultural competence include the same issues of any palliative care encounter, except that end-of-life problems may be compounded by cultural barriers and disparities. The primary (interrelated) issues include

A. *Access to care:* Health disparities and barriers lead to underutilization of services and undertreatment of patients and populations, leading, in turn, to unnecessary suffering and poorer outcomes for minorities, especially patients who are foreign-born and do not speak English (Kemp, 2005).

B. *Isolation:* Dying is often a lonely process, and more so when patients, families, and providers are unable to fully communicate with one another.

C. *Communications:* Language barriers are but one aspect of communications affecting cross-cultural communications. Other communications issues include
   1. Unspoken clues to feelings
   2. Social class barriers such as reluctance to question providers
   3. Gender barriers such as aversion to examination by a person of opposite gender or verbalization of sensitive issues such as gynecologic symptoms.

D. *Decision making:* Informed consent is based upon a relatively complete understanding of issues involved in the consent. Lack of education affects understanding of treatment, risks, and related issues; culture and religion also may play central roles in decision making (e.g., autopsy, organ donation).

E. *Spiritual distress:* Providing spiritual care can be difficult even without denominational differences. Reaching across cultural and religious barriers to provide such care is a major challenge.

Strategies to Increase and Maintain Optimal Cultural Competence

A. *Generic cultural competence* is gained through education in cross-cultural care and in providing care to people and communities from cultures other than one's own. Assessment of individual or family cultural issues related to the end of life includes the following questions that clinicians can ask patients and their loved ones to gain more understanding (Tripp-Reimer, Brink, & Saunders, 1984).
   1. What do you think caused this to happen?
   2. Do you have an explanation for why your illness started when it did?
   3. What does this sickness do to you? How does it work?
   4. How severe is this sickness? How long do you expect to live?
   5. What problems has this sickness caused you or your family?
   6. What do you fear about this sickness?
   7. What kind of treatment do you think you should receive at this point?

8. What are the most important results you hope to receive from this treatment?
9. Do you have other hopes or fears?

B. *Specific cultural competence* is gained through education on specific cultures and experience in providing care to people and communities representing the culture.
   1. Participant observation is awareness of one's interactions and the effects they have on others and is basic to deepening cultural competence.
   2. Collaboration with community groups to enhance individual and institutional competence usually is easily accomplished, as communities generally are pleased to participate in increasing understanding of their culture(s).
   3. Information on cultures in both print and electronic media has expanded exponentially in recent decades. For example, using the search engine Google (www.google.com) and inputting the terms *Vietnamese culture* or *Vietnamese health* quickly leads to links to valuable information on EthnoMed, Baylor University, and other sites.

C. *Institutional cultural competence* is increased through promoting an institutional culture of openness to other cultures, promoting cultural self-assessment, educating staff on cross-cultural care, and adapting services to accommodate other cultures.

Professional Competencies

A. Institutional
   1. Identify and utilize resources to expand institutional cultural competence.
   2. Assess the community beyond people already being seen or treated at one's institution because barriers and disparities result in some cultures being "invisible" and unable to access health care.
   3. Promote the development and expansion of cultural competencies within one's institution and profession.
   4. Promote the development and expansion of evidence-based research related to or including cultural competency (Goode et al., 2006).

B. Individual (Chrisman, 2007; Deshotels, 2002; Kemp & Rasbridge, 2004)
   1. Identify and utilize resources to expand individual cultural competence.
   2. Develop and expand cultural competencies, especially related to the cultures within one's community and institution.
   3. Evaluate individual patient and family cultural preferences.
   4. Demonstrate the ability to respect, understand, and enter effectively into other people's culture and life.
   5. Provide cultural interventions that optimize quality of care.
   6. Promote the development and expansion of evidence-based research related to or including cultural competency (Goode et al., 2006).

Patient Outcomes

A. Physical, psychosocial, and spiritual human needs are met to the extent possible.

B. Optimal communication, respect, and dignity are achieved despite cultural diversity.

C. Cultural practices perceived as significant are followed and integrated into the plan of care (Deshotels, 2002).

References

Chrisman, N.J. (2007). Extending cultural competence through systems change: Academic, hospital, and community partnerships. *Journal of Transcultural Nursing, 18*(Suppl. 1), 68S–76S.

Deshotels, J.M. (2002). Cultural awareness. In K.K. Kuebler & P. Esper (Eds.), *Palliative practices from A–Z for the bedside clinician* (pp. 67–69). Pittsburgh, PA: Oncology Nursing Society.

Drew, J.C. (2006). Cultural competence: Common ground for partnerships in health care. In E.T. Anderson & J. McFarlane (Eds.), *Community as partner* (5th ed., pp. 111–313). Philadelphia: Lippincott Williams & Wilkins.

Flaskerud, J.H. (2007). Cultural competence: What is it? *Issues in Mental Health Nursing, 28,* 121–123.

Goode, T.D., Dunne, M.C., & Bronheim, S.M. (2006). The evidence base for cultural and linguistic competency in health care. *Commonwealth Fund, 37,* 1–46.

Kemp, C.E. (2005). Cultural issues in palliative care. *Seminars in Oncology Nursing, 21,* 44–52.

Kemp, C., & Rasbridge, L.A. (2004). *Refugee and immigrant health.* Cambridge, UK: Cambridge University Press.

Lo, H.T., & Fung, K.P. (2003). Culturally competent psychotherapy. *Canadian Journal of Psychiatry, 48,* 161–170.

Tripp-Reimer, T., Brink, P.J., & Saunders, J.M. (1984). Cultural assessment: Content and process. *Nursing Outlook, 32,* 78–82.

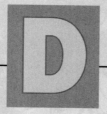

Death and Dying

Dehydration

Delirium

Depression

Diarrhea

Dyspnea

Death and Dying

Debra E. Heidrich, MSN, RN, ACHPN®, AOCN®

Definitions

Death is physiologically defined as the absence of a heartbeat and respirations. It is the expected outcome in the palliative care setting. Dying is a process that begins at birth. In the palliative care setting, the term *dying* most often refers to the final weeks, days, or hours of life.

Pathophysiology and Etiology

Many different pathophysiologic processes can lead to organ failure and eventual cessation of cardiac and respiratory function. These processes can include a direct insult to the organ from the terminal illness (e.g., respiratory failure with lung cancer) or an indirect insult to a vital system because of complications of the disease (e.g., heart block caused by hypercalcemia). When one body system fails, others also are compromised and eventually fail. As this is often a slowly progressive process in the palliative care setting, signs and symptoms of body system failure may start subtly and become more profound as death approaches.

Manifestations

A decline in functional status is often the first indication that a patient is entering the terminal phase of the disease (Gauthier, 2005). Patients who are approaching the end of life often become increasingly weak and sleepy; become less interested in getting out of bed, receiving visitors, and engaging in the activities around them; and become confused (Furst & Doyle, 2004). Symptoms the patient has been experiencing may become worse or subside as the disease progresses, and new symptoms may appear (Furst & Doyle; Mercadante, Casuccio, & Fulfaro, 2000). Frequent assessment of the patient is required to identify troublesome symptoms early and intervene to promote comfort.

A. The seven symptoms most often reported in the literature at the end of life include the following (Klinkenberg, Willems, Wal, & Deeg, 2004).

1. Fatigue
2. Pain
3. Dyspnea
4. Depression
5. Anxiety
6. Confusion
7. Nausea and/or vomiting

B. Signs and symptoms of imminent death include the following (Berry & Griffie, 2005; Ferris, von Gunten, & Emanuel, 2003; Moneymaker, 2005; Pitorak, 2003).
   1. Profound weakness
   2. Decreased level of consciousness (not universal, but common)
   3. Decreased circulation, evidenced by cool skin, mottling, and peripheral cyanosis
   4. Decreased urine output with incontinence or retention
   5. Changes in breathing patterns, including tachypnea, dyspnea, or apnea spells/Cheyne-Stokes respirations
   6. Changes in sensory perception, especially a decline in visual acuity
   7. "Nearing death awareness" experiences
      a) Nearing death awareness (Callanan & Kelley, 1992) is a special knowledge of what dying and death are like and also of what the individual needs to die peacefully. These experiences may be mistakenly labeled as "confusion."
      b) Common themes of these experiences include
         (1) Describing a place
         (2) Talking to, or being in the presence of, someone who is not alive
         (3) Knowledge of when death will occur
         (4) Choosing a time of death
         (5) Needing reconciliation
         (6) Preparing for travel or change
         (7) Being held back
         (8) Symbolic dreams.

Management

Minimal evidence-based practice exists for this topic and is included as available with each recommendation.

A. Death is anticipated in days.
   1. Treat all symptoms aggressively with the goal of comfort. (See appropriate sections for the specific symptoms.) In most circumstances, treatment of pain should not be discontinued or decreased simply because that person can no longer report pain or can no longer swallow. This will precipitate uncomfortable withdrawal.

2. Teach the family the signs and symptoms of dying, both to prepare them for the changes they will see and to assist them in recognizing when death is approaching.

3. Provide emotional and spiritual support for the patient and family using an interdisciplinary approach.

4. Anticipate the patient's needs and evaluate for any potential discomfort that the patient may not be able to communicate clearly. The profound weakness associated with the dying process can lead to anxiety and fear. Educate the family regarding these changes.

5. Evaluate medication requirements, and discontinue those that are no longer needed for medical management.

6. When the patient is not able to swallow medications, determine the best option for an alternate route of administration based on the patient's location (home versus inpatient facility), preferences, burdens associated with the alternate route, and available support systems.

   a) The gastrointestinal tract is considered the least invasive and least expensive route of medication administration.

      (1) Consult a pharmacist regarding which medications can be crushed, dissolved in water, or administered sublingually (SL) or buccally when swallowing is difficult.

      (2) Suppositories also are an option, but around-the-clock rectal administration of medications may be objectionable to the patient and family.

      (3) Some medications are available commercially in suppository form. Many medications made for oral administration appear to be effective when administered rectally for symptom management by placing the pills in a gelatin capsule. However, very little research exists to support this practice. Consult a knowledgeable pharmacist to determine the need to increase, decrease, or maintain the dose when switching to the rectal route.

   b) Subcutaneous (SC) or IV routes of administration also may be considered when the gastrointestinal tract is not an option.

7. Teach caregivers to keep the patient's mouth clean and moist.

8. Monitor for urinary incontinence, and intervene to keep skin clean and dry.

   a) Catheterization may not be required as output decreases.

   b) If turning and cleaning is uncomfortable for the dying patient or overly burdensome for the caregivers, catheterization is appropriate for the incontinent patient.

9. Monitor for urinary retention. Foley catheterization often is more comfortable than intermittent catheterization.

10. Treat the discomfort and anxiety associated with dyspnea. (See Dyspnea.)

11. Prepare the patient and family for nearing-death-awareness experiences. Some patients are reluctant to share these experiences for fear of being

labeled crazy or confused. However, these experiences often are a source of comfort for both the patient and the family.

12. Treat confusion, agitation, and restlessness appropriately. (See individual sections.)

B. Death is anticipated in hours.

1. Continue to treat physical symptoms to achieve comfort.

2. Continue to evaluate the need for medications, and discontinue as many as appropriate to maintain good symptom management. Be sure to consider the potential for withdrawal symptoms.

3. Teach the family that skin mottling, peripheral hypoxia with pale or bluish nail beds, and cool extremities are anticipated. The patient may or may not experience feeling cold. Blankets provide sufficient comfort. Heating devices (heating pads, hot-water bottles, packs heated in a microwave) should be used with caution, if at all, as the patient may not be able to perceive or articulate if the device is too hot, causing tissue damage.

4. Decrease the distress associated with noisy respirations. "Death rattle" is probably more distressing to the family than to the patient. However, hearing is believed to remain intact longer than other senses, making this potentially distressing to the patient, as well.

   a) Position changes may minimize noisy respirations. Positioning patients on their side often prevents secretions from pooling at the top of the airway.

   b) Occasionally, suctioning the upper airway can remove pooled secretions. Avoid deep suctioning; it is painful and counterproductive and stimulates more secretions. Be aware that suctioning with a Yankauer device may be uncomfortable, too, especially to patients with dyspnea (Furst & Doyle, 2004).

   c) Anticholinergic medications can be administered to reduce the production of secretions and can prevent noisy respirations (Furst & Doyle 2004; Pitorak, 2003). These agents should be used with caution because they can cause confusion and agitation. They do not affect existing secretions; early intervention is needed to prevent accumulation of secretions. Meticulous mouth care will be required to treat the dry-mouth side effect. Use of anticholinergics for this purpose is off label and is based on clinical experiences of practitioners in palliative care, not research. No studies have compared the benefits and burdens of the various anticholinergic agents used for this purpose (Furst & Doyle, 2004; Twycross & Wilcock, 2006).

      (1) Atropine 1% ophthalmic solution ($)—four drops SL every four hours, as needed

      (2) Atropine ($)—0.4–0.6 mg SC every four hours, as needed, or 1.2–2.4 mg/24 hours by continuous SC infusion

      (3) Glycopyrrolate (Robinul®) ($$)—0.2–0.4 mg SC every six hours, as needed (may have fewer central nervous system side effects, as

it does not cross the blood-brain barrier); some centers give the parenteral solution SL.

    (4) Hyoscyamine (Levsin®) ($$)—0.125–0.25 mg SL every four hours (available in solution or SL tablet)

    (5) Scopolamine transdermal patch (Transderm-Scop®) ($$)—every three days (not optimal for the imminently dying patient, as it may take several hours to achieve effect)

5. Provide emotional and spiritual support for the patient and family using the interdisciplinary team.

Patient Outcomes

A. All symptoms are optimally controlled to the time of death.

B. A peaceful death is attained.

References

Berry, P.H., & Griffie, J. (2005). Planning for the actual death. In B.R. Ferrell & N. Coyle (Eds.), *Textbook of palliative nursing* (2nd ed., pp. 561–580). New York: Oxford University Press.

Callanan, M., & Kelley, P. (1992). *Final gifts: Understanding the special awareness, needs, and communications of the dying.* New York: Bantam Books.

Ferris, F.D., von Gunten, C.F., & Emanuel, L.L. (2003). Competency in end-of-life care: Last hours of life. *Journal of Palliative Medicine, 6,* 605–613.

Furst, C.J., & Doyle, D. (2004). The terminal phase. In D. Doyle, G. Hanks, N. Cherny, & K. Calman (Eds.), *Oxford textbook of palliative medicine* (3rd ed., pp. 1119–1133). New York: Oxford University Press.

Gauthier, D.M. (2005). Decision making near the end of life. *Journal of Hospice and Palliative Nursing, 7,* 82–90.

Klinkenberg, M., Willems, D.L., Wal, G.V.D., & Deeg, D.J.H. (2004). Symptom burden in the last week of life. *Journal of Pain and Symptom Management, 27,* 5–13.

Mercadante, S., Casuccio, A., & Fulfaro, F. (2000). The course of symptom frequency and intensity in advanced cancer patients followed at home. *Journal of Pain and Symptom Management, 20,* 104–112.

Moneymaker, K.A. (2005). Understanding the dying process: Transitions during the final days to hours. *Journal of Palliative Medicine, 8,* 1079.

Pitorak, E.F. (2003). Care at the time of death. *American Journal of Nursing, 103*(7), 42–52.

Twycross, R., & Wilcock, A. (Eds.). (2006). *Hospice and palliative care formulary USA.* Nottingham, United Kingdom: Palliativedrugs.com Ltd.

Dehydration

Kim K. Kuebler, MN, RN, APRN-BC, and
Valarie A. Pompey, MS, APRN-BC, AOCNP®

Definitions

Dehydration and *volume depletion* are used interchangeably to describe the fluid deficit that interferes with normal homeostasis (Berk & Rana, 2006). Dehydration is the overall reduction of water content within the human body, particularly within the intracellular space (Sarhill, Walsh, Nelson, & Davis, 2001). Dehydration can be associated with the normal dying process, when patients begin to demonstrate a lack of interest in food and water intake, and often is a reversible component to the management of multiple symptoms.

Pathophysiology and Etiology

Dehydration reflects a shift in fluid from the intracellular to extracellular compartments in order to maintain cellular homeostasis resulting in hypernatremia (Sarhill et al., 2001). Dehydration can occur as a result of gastrointestinal losses (i.e., vomiting, diarrhea) or from persistent insensible losses (fevers) and presents as a hypernatremic, hypovolemic state (Berk & Rana, 2006). Dehydration directly affects the body's blood volume and circulatory reserve. The lack of circulatory volume influences the body's baroreceptors, contributing to multiple symptoms (e.g., dizziness, weakness, delirium). Fluid deficits, whether they are volume depletion (intravascular water and electrolytes) or dehydration (total body water deficit), place patients at risk for numerous adverse consequences, including changes in behavior, cognition, and energy level (Sarhill et al.). Dehydration can cause confusion, restlessness, and neuromuscular irritability (Fainsinger, 2002). Prolonged reduction in intravascular volume and glomerular filtration rate are known to precipitate prerenal failure (Lawlor, 2002).

Manifestations

- Opiate toxicities
- Nightmares
- Hallucinations

- Increased temperature
- Confusion
- Lethargy
- Hyperalgesia
- Constipation
- Restlessness
- Decreased jugular venous pressure
- Dry mucous membranes
- Thirst
- Myoclonus
- Fatigue
- Poor skin turgor, "tenting"
- Weakness
- Delirium
- Syncope or dizziness
- Orthostatic hypotension
- Tachycardia
- Decreased urine output

(Fainsinger, 2002; Kuebler, Heidrich, Vena, & English, 2006; Kuebler & Pompey, 2007; Lawlor, 2002)

Diagnostic Abnormalities

- Increased plasma protein
- Increased hematocrit
- Increased blood urea nitrogen and creatinine
- Increased urine osmolality
- Increased plasma sodium
- Increased or decreased plasma pH

(Berk & Rana, 2006; Dalal & Bruera, 2004; Kedziera, 2001; MacDonald, 2002; Sarhill et al., 2001)

Management

A. General measures to accomplish hydration when fluid replacement by mouth requires augmentation
   1. Parenteral infusions ($$)
   2. Proctoclysis ($) (administration of fluids rectally)
   3. Hypodermoclysis ($) (subcutaneous administration of fluids)
   (Dalal & Bruera, 2004; Fainsinger, 2002; Sarhill et al., 2001)

B. Death is not imminent.
   1. When the decision is made to hydrate a patient, various options are available.
   2. Patients should always be encouraged to take oral fluids.

3. **Level I—high level of evidence**

IV fluid replacement with crystalloid solutions (Dalal & Bruera, 2004; Fainsinger, 2002; Heitz & Horne, 2005; Kedziera, 2001; Lawlor, 2002; MacDonald, 2002; Sarhill et al., 2001)

a) Normal saline (isotonic): Expands extracellular fluid (ECF) only; does not affect intracellular fluid (ICF); used as an intravascular volume expander or to replace abnormal losses

b) Dextrose and water: Provides free water only and corrects ECF and ICF losses (to replace insensible losses and correct hypernatremia); used to treat total body water deficits only

4. **Level II—moderate level of evidence**

(Frisoli Junior, de Paula, Feldman, & Nasri, 2000; Moriarty & Hudson, 2001; Sarhill et al., 2001)

a) Proctoclysis may be a viable alternative when life expectancy is limited, as it is relatively risk free, inexpensive, and easy to administer. However, thought should be given to whether family members are willing to assume physical care associated with this approach.

b) Hypodermoclysis provides easier access; sites can last up to a week and can be easily discontinued. If subcutaneous absorption is poor, clinicians may consider adding 150–750 mcg hyaluronidase (Wydase®) to 1,000 ml normal saline.

C. Death is imminent.

1. If the patient is close to death, it may not be necessary to hydrate; this is an individual patient-specific decision.

2. However, dose adjusting is important for specific medications (e.g., opioids, anticholinergics, benzodiazepines) that can create untoward symptoms such as delirium, agitation, or myoclonus in patients who are dehydrated. Adjust the dose of specific medications to prevent drug metabolite accumulation (Dalal & Bruera, 2004; Fainsinger, 2002; Kuebler et al., 2006; Lawlor, 2002; Lawlor & Bruera, 2002; Morita, Shima, Miyashita, Kimurs, & Adachi, 2004; Sarhill et al., 2001).

Patient Outcomes

A. Optimal hydration is maintained based upon specific patient goals and preferences.

B. Symptoms resulting from dehydration are minimized.

References

Berk, L., & Rana, S. (2006). Hypovolemia and dehydration in the oncology patient. *Journal of Supportive Oncology, 4,* 447–453.

Dalal, S., & Bruera, E. (2004). Dehydration in cancer patients: To treat or not to treat. *Journal of Supportive Oncology, 2,* 467–486.

Fainsinger, R. (2002). Hydration. In C. Ripamonti & E. Bruera (Eds.), *Gastrointestinal symptoms in advanced cancer patients* (pp. 395–410). New York: Oxford University Press.

Frisoli Junior, A., de Paula, A., Feldman, D., & Nasri, F. (2000). Subcutaneous hydration by hypodermoclysis: A practical and low cost treatment for elderly patients. *Drugs and Aging, 16,* 313–319.

Heitz, U., & Horne, M. (Eds.). (2005). *Pocket guide to fluid, electrolyte and acid-base balance* (5th ed.). St. Louis, MO: Elsevier Mosby.

Kedziera, P. (2001). Hydration, thirst, and nutrition. In B.R. Ferrell & N. Coyle (Eds.), *Textbook of palliative nursing* (pp. 156–163). New York: Oxford University Press.

Kuebler, K., Heidrich, D., Vena, C., & English, N. (2006). Delirium, confusion and agitation. In B. Ferrell & N. Coyle (Eds.), *Textbook of palliative nursing* (2nd ed., pp. 401–420). New York: Oxford University Press.

Kuebler, K., & Pompey, V. (2007). Dehydration. In K.K. Kuebler, D.E. Heidrich, & P. Esper (Eds.), *Palliative and end-of-life care: Clinical practice guidelines* (2nd ed., pp. 315–325). St. Louis, MO: Elsevier Saunders.

Lawlor, P. (2002). Delirium and dehydration: Some fluid for thought? *Supportive Care in Cancer, 10,* 445–454.

Lawlor, P., & Bruera, E. (2002). Delirium in patients with advanced cancer. *Hematology/Oncology Clinics of North America, 16,* 701–714.

MacDonald, N. (2002). Ethical considerations in feeding or hydrating advanced cancer patients. In C. Ripamonti & E. Bruera (Eds.), *Gastrointestinal symptoms in advanced cancer patients* (pp. 411–423). New York: Oxford University Press.

Moriata, T., Shima, Y., Miyashita, M., Kimurs, R., & Adachi, I. (2004). Physician and nurse reported effects of intravenous hydration therapy on symptoms of terminally ill patients with cancer. *Journal of Palliative Medicine, 7,* 683–693.

Moriarty, D., & Hudson, E. (2001). Hypodermoclysis for rehydration in the community. *British Journal of Community Nursing, 6,* 437–443.

Sarhill, N., Walsh, D., Nelson, K., & Davis, M. (2001). Evaluation and treatment of cancer-related fluid deficits: Volume depletion and dehydration. *Supportive Care in Cancer, 9,* 408–419.

Delirium

Kim K. Kuebler, MN, RN, APRN-BC, and
Valarie A. Pompey, MS, APRN-BC, AOCNP®

Definition

Delirium is defined as an acute confused state that results from a diffuse organic brain dysfunction. Delirium is one of the most difficult syndromes to diagnose and treat, and it substantially interfaces with a decline in quality of life for the patient and the observing family in the dying phase (Centeno, Sanz, & Bruera, 2004). Delirium is a major cause for admission into palliative care units and often is characterized by an acute state of confusion with varied manifestations that fluctuate over time, thus increasing the complexity of symptom recognition (Centeno et al.; Morrisson, 2003). Delirium often is characterized by the concurrent disturbance in the level of consciousness and deficits in attention, orientation, sleep-wake cycles, thinking, and memory (Boyle, 2006; Centeno et al.; Greenberg, 2003). Key findings that help to distinguish delirium from dementia are the fluctuating nature of its clinical presentation (Boyle; Centeno et al.; Greenberg) and its sudden, abrupt onset (Boyle; Centeno et al.; Jackson & Lipman, 2004; Kress & Hall, 2004).

Pathophysiology and Etiology

Common in patients with advanced cancer, delirium can occur in as many as 25%–40% of patients and in as many as 85% of those who are actively dying (Boyle, 2006; Centeno et al., 2004; Lawlor & Bruera, 2002; Ross & Alexander, 2001). The exact pathophysiology is not well understood, but delirium can be precipitated by myriad factors and is considered reversible in the majority of cases (Boyle; Centeno et al.; Vena, 2007). Because very little is known about delirium's underlying pathophysiology, the diagnosis of delirium is primarily clinical and based upon careful observation and awareness of key features (Clary & Krishnan, 2001). The clinician should evaluate the patient for a constellation of findings that include subtle changes or disturbances of consciousness and/or changes in cognition (Kuebler, Heidrich, Vena, & English, 2006).

The authors would like to acknowledge Howard Smith, MD, for his contribution that remains unchanged from the first edition of this textbook.

Two explanatory models for delirium have been developed to identify precipitating factors that lead to delirium (Breitbart & Cohen, 2000). In the first model, delirium is viewed as a global and nonspecific disorder of the brain and characterized by a generalized dysfunction in cerebral metabolism. The second model suggests that derangements in specific neurotransmitter systems precipitate brain pathology. Delirium is most likely a symptom of a variety of disorders that feature specific or multiple interacting neurotransmitter systems impairment as a result of aberrant metabolic activity, hypoxia, or exogenous agents (Samuels & Neugroschl, 2005).

A. Predisposing factors of delirium include
   1. Older age
   2. Male gender
   3. Drug or alcohol dependence
   4. Frailty
   5. Impairments in perception (vision, hearing)
   6. Poor nutritional status
   7. Insufficient sleep/dreams
   8. Depression
   9. Chronic advanced illness (organ failure).

B. Precipitating factors of delirium include (Boyle, 2006; Centeno et al., 2004; Clary & Krishnan, 2001; Jackson & Lipman, 2004; Vena, 2007)
   1. Immobility (restraints)
   2. Unfamiliar surroundings
   3. Sensory overload or deprivation
   4. Intensive care unit admission
   5. Metabolic abnormalities (hypercalcemia, uremia)
   6. Anemia
   7. Hypoxemia
   8. Sepsis/infection
   9. Symptoms (pain, urinary retention, constipation, dyspnea).

C. Additional considerations include
   1. Electrolyte imbalance (dehydration)
   2. Brain tumors, central nervous system (CNS) metastasis, and other CNS disorders such as stroke
   3. Seizure disorders
   4. Drugs (opioids, steroids, benzodiazepines, anticholinergics)
   5. Cardiopulmonary abnormalities
   6. Trauma
   7. Environment
   8. Paraneoplastic syndromes
   9. Fever.

Manifestations

Delirium differs in its presentation among patients, and symptoms frequently fluctuate, making it difficult to detect. Because of the difficulty in assessing delirium, it can often go undiagnosed (Inouye, Foreman, Mion, & Cooney, 2001).

Patients in the early stages of delirium can be asymptomatic. Symptoms vary from patient to patient and can fluctuate in the same patient from day to day (Boyle, 2006; Centeno et al., 2004). Prodromal symptoms are often subtle and typically are attributed to other causes (Boyle). Manifestations of delirium include the following.

- Confused thinking
- Forgetfulness
- Difficulty concentrating
- Difficulty judging the passing of time
- Feeling "mixed up" or "fuzzy"
- Perceptual distortions

Behavioral manifestations of anxiety, unusual restlessness, irritability, disturbances in mood, withdrawal, hypersensitivity to light and noise, insomnia and daytime sleepiness, and vivid dreams can occur. A single nocturnal episode of confusion can be observed and sometimes is diagnosed as depression or dementia (Boyle, 2006).

Delirium can be further categorized as being *hyperactive, hypoactive,* or *mixed.*

- *Hyperactive:* The patient is restless and aroused but cannot sustain attention. This often is associated with liver failure, dehydration, opioid toxicity, or aggressive steroid therapy.
- *Hypoactive:* The patient is drowsy, and the clinician may have difficulty in generating attention. This often is caused by a condition such as dehydration, medication toxicities (i.e., dioxin), or hypoglycemia and can be mistaken for depression or fatigue (Boyle, 2006; Centeno et al., 2004; Hoofring, Olsen, & Taylor, 2007).
- *Mixed:* The patient experiences a combination of hyperactive and hypoactive symptoms.

Management

The following interventions are considered for the care and management of the dying patient.

A. Pharmacologic interventions
   1. When considering the pharmacologic management of delirium, the clinician must consider the issue of disease presentation (Jackson & Lipman, 2004). Currently, controlled trials of pharmacology use in the management of delirium that are differentiated by type of delirium (i.e., hyperactive and hypoactive) are limited. A recent Cochrane review identified one controlled trial that was considered evidence appropriate, and this paper identified

the use of haloperidol in the management of delirium in the dying patient population (Jackson & Lipman).

2. **Level II—moderate level of evidence**
   Neuroleptics (butyrophenones)
   a) Haloperidol (Haldol®) ($)—0.5–5 mg every four hours/max 20 mg per 24 hours.
   b) Haloperidol is considered the pharmacotherapy of choice for delirium in the dying patient and has been shown to be effective in the management of the three types of delirium. It is the least sedating and can be administered po, IV, intramuscular, or subcutaneous.

3. **Level III—low level of evidence**
   (Boyle, 2006; Centeno et al., 2004; Greenberg, 2003; Jackson & Lipman, 2004; Lawlor & Bruera, 2002; Ross & Alexander, 2001)
   a) Chlorpromazine (Thorazine®) ($)—25 mg every eight hours. Similar efficacy as haloperidol; minimal extrapyramidal effects in low doses.
   b) Benzodiazepines
      (1) Lorazepam (Ativan®) ($$)—Sedating with treatment-related side effects common over time (e.g., agitation)
      (2) Midazolam ($$)—Used when rapid sedation is needed, until the underlying cause of delirium is found; has short half-life and is quickly reversible
   c) Neuroleptics (thienobenzodiazepines)
      (1) Olanzapine (Zyprexa®) ($$)—2.5 mg–5 mg at bedtime
      (2) Risperidone (Risperdal®) ($$)—0.25 mg–0.5 mg bid
      (3) Both have been recommended for short-term use of a week or less, are not available in IV form, and have not been specifically studied in delirium.

B. Nonpharmacologic interventions
   Level III—low level of evidence
   1. Identify and reverse possible causes.
      a) Drugs (opioid rotation, taper other drugs as needed)
      b) Dehydration (fluid and electrolyte replacement)
      c) Infection (antibiotics)
      d) Metabolic abnormalities (fluid and electrolyte replacement)
      e) Hypoxia (oxygen or blood product replacement as needed)
   2. Take preventive measures.
      a) Provide a calm, quiet environment.
      b) Limit changes in routine.
      c) Limit sensory stimulus.

Patient Outcomes

A. Symptom distress is decreased.

B. Patient experiences comfort and cognition when interacting with others.

C. Safety is maintained.

References

Boyle, D.A. (2006). Delirium in older adults with cancer: Implications for practice and research. *Oncology Nursing Forum, 33,* 61–78.

Breitbart, W., & Cohen, K. (2000). Delirium in the terminally ill. In H.M. Chochinov & W. Breitbart (Eds.), *Handbook of psychiatry in palliative medicine* (pp. 75–90). New York: Oxford University Press.

Centeno, C., Sanz, A., & Bruera, E. (2004). Delirium in advanced cancer patients. *Palliative Medicine, 18,* 184–194.

Clary, G., & Krishnan, K. (2001). Delirium: Diagnosis, neuropathogenesis, and treatment. *Journal of Psychiatric Practice, 7,* 310–323.

Greenberg, D.B. (2003). Preventing delirium at the end of life: Lessons from recent research. *Primary Care Companion, Journal of Clinical Psychiatry, 5,* 62–67.

Hoofring, L., Olsen, M., & Taylor, K. (2007). Management of delirium—case study. *Oncology, 21,* 29–31.

Inouye, S.K., Foreman, M.D., Mion, L.C., & Cooney, L.M., Jr. (2001). Nurses' recognition of delirium and its symptoms: Comparison of nurse and researcher ratings. *Archives of Internal Medicine, 161,* 2467–2473.

Jackson, K.C., & Lipman, A.G. (2004). Drug therapy for delirium in terminally ill patients. *Cochrane Database of Systematic Reviews 2004,* Issue 2. Art. No.: CD004770. DOI: 10.1002/14651858. CD004770.

Kress, J.P., & Hall, J.B. (2004). Delirium and sedation. *Critical Care Clinics, 20,* 419–433.

Kuebler, K., Heidrich, D., Vena, C., & English, N. (2006). Delirium, confusion, and agitation. In B. Ferrell & N. Coyle (Eds.), *Textbook of palliative nursing* (2nd ed., pp. 401–420). New York: Oxford University Press.

Lawlor, P.G., & Bruera, E.D. (2002). Delirium in patients with advanced cancer. *Hematology/Oncology Clinics of North America, 16,* 701–714.

Morrisson, C. (2003). Identification and management of delirium in the critically ill patient with cancer. *AACN Critical Issues, 14,* 92–111.

Ross, D.D., & Alexander, C.S. (2001). Management of common symptoms in terminally ill patients: Part II. Constipation, delirium and dyspnea. *American Family Physician, 64,* 1019–1026.

Samuels, S., & Neugroschl, J. (2005). Delirium. In B. Sadock & V. Sadock (Eds.), *Kaplan & Sadock's comprehensive textbook of psychiatry* (8th ed., pp. 1054–1067). Philadephia: Lippincott Williams & Wilkins.

Vena, C. (2007). Delirium and acute confusion. In K.K. Kuebler, D.E. Heidrich, & P. Esper (Eds.), *Palliative and end-of-life care: Clinical practice guidelines* (2nd ed., pp. 327–348). St. Louis, MO: Elsevier Saunders.

Depression

Shawn D. Salkow, PharmD

Definition

Depression is a mood state that spans a continuum from minor alterations in mood to pathologic loss of the ability to cope with life. It is recognized as the most common mental health problem in palliative care.

Pathophysiology and Etiology

Advanced illness can produce many of the somatic signs and symptoms (e.g., difficulty sleeping, poor appetite, loss of energy, reduced concentration) seen in depression (Block, 2000). A diagnosis of depression in advanced cancer is based on psychological or cognitive symptoms (e.g., worthlessness, hopelessness, excessive guilt, suicidal ideation) of major depression (American Psychiatric Association [APA], 2000a). After being diagnosed with a terminal illness (e.g., late-stage cancer, HIV), the patient begins to have a decreased drive to live. Depression is eight times more prevalent in terminally ill patients with a desire for death compared to terminally ill patients without a significant desire for death (Chochinov et al., 1995). Conventional treatment leads to a positive response in more than 80% of cases. However, evidence suggests that many cases of depression are not diagnosed (Breitbart, Chochinov, & Passik, 1998).

Manifestations

- Depressed mood is reported or observed to be distinctly different from normal mood variations and causes suffering, distress, or dysfunction.
- Depressed mood is present most of the day for at least two weeks.
- Sadness may be part of a normal adjustment reaction and may require counseling and social support rather than medication. Symptoms that meet diagnostic

The author would like to acknowledge William Breitbart, MD, E. Duke Dickerson, MSc, PhD, John L. Shuster, Jr., MD, Jeffery P. Henderson, MS, Joshua M. Cox, RPh, and Mellar P. Davis, MD, FCCP, for their contributions that remain unchanged from the first edition of this textbook.

criteria should be treated with antidepressant medications and augmented by counseling and social contact.

Barriers to Diagnosis

Three possible explanations for underrecognizing and misdiagnosing depression are
- Patients and clinicians believe psychological distress to be a normal feature of the dying process.
- Many clinicians lack the expertise to differentiate among depression, anxiety, and delirium in terminally ill patients.
- Many patients and clinicians are unwilling to consider a diagnosis of clinical depression because of the negative connotation associated with the diagnosis of of a life-limited illness (Block, 2000).

Management

A. Death is not imminent (i.e., patients with a life expectancy of more than four weeks).
1. **Level I—high level of evidence**
   Pharmacologic interventions (APA, 2000b; Furukawa, McGuire, & Barburi, 2003)
   a) Selective serotonin reuptake inhibitors (SSRIs) ($–$$$)
      (1) Citalopram (Celexa®)—initially 20 mg po daily, generally with an increase to 40 mg*
      (2) Escitalopram (Lexapro®)—10 mg po daily.* May be increased to 20 mg po daily. 20 mg failed to demonstrate greater benefit compared to 10 mg.
      (3) Fluoxetine
         (a) Prozac®—20 mg po every morning* is the recommended starting dose. The dose may be increased by 20 mg intervals to a maximum of 80 mg daily if insufficient clinical improvement is reached within several weeks. Each dose increase should spaced by a minimum of one to two weeks.
         (b) Prozac Weekly—The dose ranges are the same as the daily option. However, the dose should only be taken on the same day once per week (i.e., every Monday) instead of daily.
      (4) Paroxetine
         (a) Paxil®—The recommended starting dose is 20 mg po every morning* This dose may be increased by 10 mg intervals to a maximum of 50 mg daily if insufficient clinical improvement is reached. Allow one week between dose increases.
         (b) Paxil CR—The recommended starting dose is 25 mg po every morning. The dose may be increased by 12.5 mg intervals to

a maximum of 62.5 mg daily if insufficient clinical improvement is reached. Allow one week between dose increases.

    (5) Sertraline (Zoloft®)—The recommended starting dose is 50 mg po daily. The dose may be increased to a maximum of 200 mg daily if insufficient clinical improvement is reached.* Allow at least one week between dose increases.

  b) Serotonin and noradrenaline reuptake inhibitors (SNRIs) ($$-$$$)

    (1) Venlafaxine (Effexor® XR and IR)—The recommended starting dose is 75 mg po daily.* The dose may be increased to a maximum of 225 mg daily if insufficient clinical improvement is reached. Allow a minimum of four days to increase the dose. The dose was increased in two-week periods in clinical trials.

    (2) Duloxetine (Cymbalta®)—The recommended starting dose is 30 mg po daily for one week, then increase to 60 mg or 40 mg (20 mg po bid); can be increased to 60 mg daily.* A dosage of 120 mg was studied in clinical trials, but no evidence exists that doses greater than 60 mg have any benefit.

  c) Low-dose tricyclic antidepressants ($)—Start at 25–50 mg po once daily, but dose should only be increased to 75–100 mg/day.*

    (1) Amitriptyline (Elavil®)

    (2) Imipramine (Tofranil®)

    (3) Nortriptyline (Pamelor®)

  2. **Level III—low level of evidence**

    Nonpharmacologic interventions

    a) Although no data are available to support exercise as an effective treatment in severe depression, data suggest it has a favorable effect on mood and sleep patterns (Porter, Linsley, & Ferrier, 2001).

    b) The level of exercise will vary from patient to patient, but each patient should be encouraged to participate in physical activity at least once a day.

    c) See Complementary and Alternative Medicine and Integrative Medicine for additional nonpharmacologic interventions.

B. **Death is imminent.**

  1. For patients with a life expectancy of four weeks or less, a psychostimulant is generally recommended.

  2. **Level II—moderate level of evidence**

    (Bukberg, Penman, & Holland, 1984; Rozans, Dreisbach, Lertora, & Kahn, 2002; Shuster, Chochinov, & Greenberg, 2000)

    a) Methylphenidate (Ritalin®) ($)—5 mg po in the morning and may be administered four hours later (e.g., 8 am and noon).*

Please note that the dosing included in the text is only a recommendation. Medication dosing must account for patient-specific characteristics including, but not limited to, age, gender, body weight (i.e., actual versus ideal), kidney function, liver function, comorbidities, existing medication regimen, and medication history. When starting a patient on a particular antidepressant, take the aforementioned characteristics into consideration when selecting an agent and strength.

    b) Dextroamphetamine (Dexedrine®) ($)—5 mg po in the morning and increased as tolerated. Maximum doses are 40–60 mg/day.*

  3. A Cochrane protocol of psychostimulants for the treatment of depression was published online July 18, 2007. This review may be published in 2008.

Measurement Instruments

A. Hospital anxiety and depression scale (HADS) (Zigmond & Snaith, 1983)
  1. This tool can be useful in identifying depressive disorders in patients with advanced illness.
  2. HADS, a 14-item self-rating questionnaire with subscales for depression and anxiety, has been demonstrated to be effective for screening depressive disorders in patients with cancer (Derogatis & Melisaratos, 1983).

B. Distress thermometer (a visual analog scale to measure nonspecific distress)

C. Prime-MD mood module (structured interview that allows accurate diagnosis of mood disorders in less than five minutes) (Spitzer et al., 1994)

Patient Outcomes

A. Target symptoms are resolved.

B. Patient experiences relief from suffering, distress, and dysfunction related to mood.

References

American Psychiatric Association. (2000a). *Diagnostic and statistical manual of mental disorders* (4th ed., text rev.). Washington, DC: Author.

American Psychiatric Association. (2000b). *Treating major depressive disorder: A quick reference guide.* Retrieved August 10, 2007, from http://www.psych.org/psych_pract/treatg/quick_ref_guide/MDD_QRG.pdf

Block, S. (2000). Assessing and managing depression in the terminally ill patient: ACP-ASIM End-of-Life Care Consensus Panel—American College of Physicians, American Society of Internal Medicine. *Annals of Internal Medicine, 132,* 209–218.

Breitbart, W., Chochinov, H., & Passik, S. (1998). Psychiatric aspects of palliative care. In D. Doyle, G.W.C. Hanks, & N. MacDonald (Eds.), *Oxford textbook of palliative medicine* (2nd ed., pp. 933–954). New York: Oxford University Press.

Bukberg, J., Penman, D., & Holland, J.C. (1984). Depression in hospitalized cancer patients. *Psychosomatic Medicine, 46,* 199–212.

Chochinov, H.M., Wilson, K.G., Enns, M., Mowchun, N., Lander, S., Levitt, M., et al. (1995). Desire for death in the terminally ill. *American Journal of Psychiatry, 152,* 1185–1191.

Derogatis, L.R., & Melisaratos, N. (1983). The brief symptom inventory (BSI): An introductory report. *Psychological Medicine, 13,* 595–605.

Furukawa, T., McGuire, H., & Barburi, C. (2003). Low dosage tricyclic antidepressants for depression. *Cochrane Database of Systematic Reviews 2003,* Issue 3. Art. No.: CD003197. DOI: 10.1002.14651858. CD003197.

Porter, R., Linsley, K., & Ferrier, N. (2001). Treatment of severe depression: Nonpharmacologic aspects. *Advances in Psychiatric Treatment, 7,* 117–124.

Rozans, M., Dreisbach, A., Lertora, J., & Kahn, M.J. (2002). Palliative uses of methylphenidate in patients with cancer: A review. *Journal of Clinical Oncology, 20,* 335–339.

Shuster, J.L., Chochinov, H.M., & Greenberg, D.B. (2000). Psychiatric aspects and psychopharmacologic strategies in palliative care. In A. Stoudemire, B.S. Fogel, & D.B. Greenberg (Eds.), *Psychiatric care of the medical patient: Vol. 2* (2nd ed., pp. 315–327). New York: Oxford University Press.

Spitzer, R.L., Williams, J.B., Kroenke, K., Linzer, M., deGruy, F.V., III, Hahn, S.R., et al. (1994). Utility of a new procedure for diagnosing mental disorders in primary care: The PRIME-MD 1000 study. *JAMA, 272,* 1749–1756.

Zigmond, A., & Snaith, R. (1983). The hospital anxiety and depression scale. *Acta Psychiatrica Scandinavica, 67,* 361–370.

Diarrhea

Debra E. Heidrich, MSN, RN, ACHPN®, AOCN®

Definition

Diarrhea is defined as an increase in stool volume and liquidity, resulting in the passage of three or more loose or unformed stools per day (Rogers, 2005; Sykes, 2004). Uncontrolled diarrhea can lead to fluid and electrolyte imbalances, resulting in lethargy, weakness, and orthostatic hypotension. Persistent diarrhea may lead to malnutrition, impaired skin integrity, altered sleeping patterns, social isolation, anxiety, and self-concept disturbances (Heidrich, 2007).

Pathophysiology and Etiology

Any condition that increases secretion within the gastrointestinal (GI) tract, interferes with reabsorption from the GI tract, increases the motility of the GI tract, or causes excretion of mucus, fluids, or blood can cause diarrhea (Lingappa, 2003; Mercadante, 2002; Sykes, 2004).

A. Conditions that increase secretions in the GI tract include
   1. Inflammation—radiation enteritis, chemotherapy, infection
   2. Infection—many types, including *Cryptosporidium sp.* and *Clostridium difficile (C. difficile),* cause profound diarrhea.
   3. Irritation—inability to absorb bile salts (e.g., because of ileal resection, gastrectomy).

B. Causes of osmotic diarrhea include excessive amounts of any of the following in the GI tract.
   1. Nonabsorbable sugars—lactulose, sorbitol
   2. Salts—magnesium, bile salts
   3. Fats—biliary obstruction, lack of pancreatic enzymes

The author would like to acknowledge Beth Cohen, RNC, ARNP, MSN, for her contribution that remains unchanged from the first edition of this textbook.

C. Hypermotility of the GI tract occurs when peristaltic activity is stimulated by
   1. Irritation—food poisoning, infections, ulcerative colitis
   2. Medications—laxatives, cholinergics (e.g., metoclopramide).

D. Exudative diarrhea occurs when excessive proteins, bleeding, or irritation are present, causing excessive mucus production.
   1. Excessive proteins—bowel obstruction
   2. Bleeding—bowel tumors, GI ulceration
   3. Excessive mucus—stimulated by an irritation caused by tumors, impaction, or bowel obstruction

Manifestations

- More than four stools per day
- Abdominal pain or cramping
- Anorectal pain or irritation
- Fluid or electrolyte imbalance
- Postural hypotension
- Fatigue or malaise
- Fever
- Anorexia
- Weakness

Management

A. Death is not imminent.
   1. Pharmacologic interventions
      a) **Level I—high level of evidence**
         (1) A quinolone antibiotic ($$$) should be prescribed for infectious diarrhea in patients who have prolonged diarrhea or who are at high risk for complications, such as older adults, diabetics, cirrhotics, and immunocompromised patients. However, routine empirical use of antibiotics is avoided because of the self-limiting nature of most cases of diarrhea, the cost of antibiotics, and the potential to worsen the problem of antibiotic resistance of enteric pathogens (Oldfield, 2001).
         (2) Antidiarrheal medications are helpful for mild to moderate chemotherapy-induced diarrhea (Cascinu et al., 2000).
            (a) Loperamide (Imodium®) ($)—4 mg po initially, followed by 2 mg after each loose stool; maximum dose 16 mg/day
            (b) Diphenoxylate (Lomotil®) ($$)—5 mg po initially, followed by 2.5–5 mg four times daily
            (c) Tincture of opium ($)—0.3–1 ml of 10% solution four times daily (5–16 drops four times a day)
                 (Note: Do not confuse tincture of opium with paregoric. Paregoric is dosed as 0.4 mg/1 ml, and tincture of opium contains

the equivalent of morphine 10 mg/1 ml. Overdose can result if not dosed in drops.)

(3) Octreotide (Sandostatin®) ($$$$) is helpful for moderate to severe chemotherapy-induced diarrhea (Major et al., 2004; Sykes, 2004). Start with 100 mcg subcutaneous three times daily and escalate every eight hours by 50–100 mcg until the diarrhea is controlled, to a maximum of 500 mcg three times daily.

b) **Level II—moderate level of evidence**

(1) Psyllium products (e.g., Metamucil®) ($) can improve stool consistency by absorbing water, decreasing the "watery" nature of the stool.

(2) Clonidine ($–$$) may be helpful for some secretory diarrheas, but the side effects of hypotension and sedation limit its usefulness (Mercadante, 2002).

2. Nonpharmacologic interventions

a) **Level II—moderate level of evidence**

Hydration—Used to prevent dehydration and electrolyte imbalance. Most instances of diarrhea in the palliative care setting are rarely of sufficient amount or duration to require hydration, with the exception of the diarrhea associated with AIDS and *C. difficile* (Sykes, 2004).

(1) Oral hydration ($–$$) is preferred, when tolerated. Options for oral hydration include

(a) Commercial sports drinks with glucose, electrolytes, and water (e.g., Gatorade®)

(b) Rehydration solutions available from pharmacies (e.g., Pedia-lyte®)

(d) A solution of 2 g (~ ½ teaspoon) salt plus 50 g (~ 4 tablespoons) sugar in one liter of water; may flavor with lemon juice (Waller & Caroline, 2000). Homemade solutions should be used within 24 hours of preparation.

(2) IV or hypodermoclysis ($$–$$$) replacement may be required if the patient is unable to tolerate sufficient oral intake.

b) **Level III—low level of evidence**

(1) Skin care ($–$$)—Steps must be taken to prevent skin breakdown.

(a) Avoid the use of diapers.

(b) Keep skin clean by using a pH-balanced cleanser or warm water. Avoid soaps, as they are drying. Avoid rubbing the area; use of a squeeze bottle with warm water may assist with cleansing.

(c) Apply a moisture barrier that contains zinc oxide, dimethicone, or silicone. Petroleum-based products should be avoided because they need to be reapplied frequently (Fleck, 2005).

(d) Consider a fecal incontinence collector if the patient is experiencing massive amounts of diarrhea to protect the skin, decrease caregiver burden, and control odor.

    i) Collection bags ($–$$)—Almost always able to use in men; in women, feasibility is determined by the skin bridge between the anus and vagina. It may be difficult to apply a pouch to severely denuded skin. Area may need to be shaved prior to applying the pouch. Skin preparation with application of a protective barrier solution is necessary.

    ii) Bowel management systems (e.g., Zassi®) ($$$)—Follow manufacturer's instructions for insertion, irrigation, and maintenance.

  (2) Dietary guidelines—Dietary alterations to help to resolve diarrhea may include following a BRATT diet: bananas, rice, applesauce, toast (plain), and tea. Avoid spicy, greasy, or gas-producing foods.

B. Death is imminent.
1. Attempts should be made, if appropriate, to treat diarrhea.
2. Keeping the patient clean, dry, and comfortable is the priority.
3. Use antidiarrheal medications, as tolerated.
4. Monitor hydration status to prevent overhydrating patients at the end of life, as retaining too much fluid appears to be more uncomfortable than being slightly dehydrated.

Patient Outcomes

A. Diarrhea is controlled.

B. Diarrhea-associated symptoms (e.g., fatigue, dehydration) are relieved, and diarrhea-associated problems are prevented.

References

Cascinu, S., Bichisao, E., Amadori, D., Silingardi, V., Giordani, P., Sansoni, E., et al. (2000). High-dose loperamide in the treatment of 5-fluorouracil-induced diarrhea in colorectal cancer patients. *Supportive Care in Cancer, 8,* 65–67.

Fleck, C.A. (2005). Ethical wound management for the palliative care patient. *Extended Care Product News, 100*(4), 38–46.

Heidrich, D.E. (2007). Diarrhea. In K.K. Kuebler, D.E. Heidrich, & P. Esper (Eds.), *Palliative and end-of-life care: Clinical practice guidelines* (2nd ed., pp. 361–376). St. Louis, MO: Elsevier Saunders.

Lingappa, V.R. (2003). Gastrointestinal disease. In S.J. McPhee, V.R. Lingappa, & W.F. Ganong (Eds.), *Pathophysiology of disease: An introduction to clinical medicine* (4th ed., pp. 340–379). New York: Lange Medical Books/McGraw-Hill.

Major, P., Figueredo, A., Tandan, V., Bramwell, V., Charette, M., & Oliver, T. (2004). *The role of octreotide in the management of patients with cancer.* Practice guideline report number 12-7. Retrieved December 21, 2007, from http://www.cancercare.on.ca/pdf/pebc12-7s.pdf

Mercadante, W. (2002). Diarrhea, malabsorption, and constipation. In A. Berger, R. Portenoy, & D. Weissman (Eds.), *Principles and practice of supportive oncology* (2nd ed., pp. 233–249). Philadelphia: Lippincott Williams & Wilkins.

Oldfield, E.C. (2001). The role of antibiotics in the treatment of infectious diarrhea. *Gastroenterology Clinics of North America, 30,* 817–836.

Rogers, H.M. (2005). Management of clients with intestinal disorders. In J.M. Black & J.H. Hawks (Eds.), *Medical-surgical nursing: Clinical management for positive outcomes* (7th ed., pp. 807–855). St. Louis, MO: Elsevier Saunders.

Sykes, N. (2004). Constipation and diarrhea. In D. Doyle, G. Hanks, N. Cherny, & K. Calman (Eds.), *Oxford textbook of palliative medicine* (3rd ed., pp. 483–496). New York: Oxford University Press.

Waller, A., & Caroline, N.L. (2000). *Handbook of palliative care in cancer* (2nd ed.). Boston: Butterworth-Heinemann.

Dyspnea

Jerald M. Andry, PharmD, MSc

Definition

The word *dyspnea* is derived from two Greek words meaning *difficult* and *breathing*. It is a sensory awareness of one's own labored breathing. Dyspnea is defined broadly by the American Thoracic Society (1999) as a subjective experience of breathing discomfort that consists of qualitatively distinct sensations that vary in intensity. The experience derives from interactions among multiple physiologic, psychological, social, and environmental factors and may induce secondary physiologic and behavioral responses.

Pathophysiology and Etiology

Dyspnea is caused by complex interactions between peripheral and central sensory receptors as well as cognition. Physiologic, psychological, behavioral, social, and environmental factors play a role in the pathogenesis and perception of dyspnea (Rao & Gray, 2003). Although the underlying medical condition may not be treatable in the palliative care patient, dyspnea almost always responds to intervention or treatment.

Dyspnea is predominantly experienced by patients with pulmonary, cardiac, and neuromuscular diseases (Waller & Caroline, 2000). Figure 18-1 summarizes some of the specific causes of dyspnea.

Manifestations

- Tachypnea
- Cyanosis
- Digital clubbing
- Memory or concentration difficulties
- Pallor

The author would like to acknowledge Pamela Spencer, BA, MSN, BSN, FNP, for her contribution that remains unchanged from the first edition of this textbook.

- Crackles or wheezing noises
- Confusion
- Intercostal retractions
- Coughing
- Use of accessory muscles
- Tachycardia
- Restlessness

(Kuebler, Andry, & Davis, 2007; Pereira & Bruera, 1997; Waller & Caroline, 2000)

Management

The goal of treatment for dyspnea is to control breathlessness, decrease anxiety, and treat the underlying etiology. The pharmacologic management is based on the etiology of this symptom. Morphine is the most commonly used medication to control dyspnea in the palliative care setting. Usually, the dose of morphine required to relieve dyspnea is less than what is needed to reduce pain, an important

---

Figure 18-1. Causes of Dyspnea

Unrelated to Cancer
- Anxiety/hyperventilation syndrome
- Arrhythmias
- Aspiration
- Asthma
- Cardiovascular disease
- Chronic obstructive pulmonary disease
- Gastroesophageal reflux disease
- Hypo- or hyperthyroidism
- Hypoxia
- Neuromuscular disorders
- Obesity
- Pneumothorax
- Pulmonary vascular disease
- Sarcoidosis
- Sepsis
- Vocal cord dysfunction

Indirectly Related to Cancer
- Anemia
- Ascites
- Cachexia
- Electrolyte imbalance
- Pleural effusion
- Pulmonary embolus
- Respiratory infection/pneumonia

Related to Cancer
- Lymphangitic tumor
- Malignant pleural infusion
- Pericardial effusion
- Pleural tumor
- Superior vena cava syndrome
- Tracheal esophageal fistula
- Tumors of the trachea, larynx, thyroid, mediastinum, or bronchus

Related to Cancer Therapy
- Chemotherapy
- Radiation
- Surgery

Note. Based on information from American Thoracic Society, 1999; Dudgeon, 2005; Jantarakupt & Porock, 2005; Thomas & von Gunten, 2003; Wickham, 1998.

consideration in patients who are not already taking opioids for pain. A systematic review of 18 studies on the use of opioids in the management of dyspnea was conducted (Jennings, Davies, Higgins, Gibbs, & Broadley, 2002). The authors concluded that the use of opioids in the treatment of breathlessness has a significant positive effect. In addition, oral or parenteral opioids showed a greater effect than nebulized formulations. A recent meta-analysis by Joyce, McSweeney, Carrieri-Kohlman, and Hawkins (2004) evaluated 20 papers for the use of nebulized opioids in treating dyspnea. Most of the sample sizes were small, and the authors concluded that not enough data are available to recommend nebulized opioids for dyspnea (Joyce et al.).

Many nonpharmacologic strategies currently are available for managing dyspnea, including breathing and relaxation techniques, body positioning, and environmental conditioning. Pursed lipped and diaphragmatic breathing techniques allow patients to decrease the amount of air that is trapped in the lungs, increase the amount of air consumed with each breath, and improve gas exchange in the lungs (Jantarakupt & Porock, 2005). Dyspneic patients who are taught to sit in the "tripod" position can find relief. This position allows the abdominal wall to move outward, increasing transdiaphragmatic pressure and allowing for more space for lung expansion and gas exchange (Sharp, Drutz, Moisan, Foster, & Machnach, 1980). Environmentally, dry, cold air can worsen dyspnea. Patients should be taught to breathe through the mouth to warm and humidify the air before it reaches the trachea (Dudgeon, 2005). Relaxation techniques that decrease anxiety are important to decrease respiratory rate and assist in controlling dyspnea (Jantarakupt & Porock). Other methods with controversial evidence to relieve dyspnea include acupuncture, massage, and hypnosis.

A. Death is not imminent.
   1. **Level I—high level of evidence**
      (Allard, Lamontagne, Bernard, & Tremblay, 1999; Bruera, Macmillan, Pither, & MacDonald, 1990; Jennings et al., 2002; Mazzocato, Buclin, & Rapin, 1999; Thomas & von Gunten, 2003; Wickham, 1998)
      a) Nonpharmacologic management, including relaxation and breathing techniques
      b) Bronchodilators ($–$$)
         (1) Nebulized
            (a) Ipratropium (Atrovent®)
            (b) Albuterol (Proventil®)
            (c) Isoproterenol (Isuprel®)
            (d) Metoproterenol (Alupent®)
            (e) Ipratropium/albuterol (DuoNeb®)
         (2) Long-acting non-nebulized agents
            (a) Tiotropium (Spiriva®)
            (b) Salmeterol (Serevent®)
            (c) Formoterol (Foradil®)
         (3) Systemic bronchodilators—theophylline (Theo-Dur®)

   c) Corticosteroids ($–$$)
     (1) Nebulized beclomethasone
     (2) Inhaled non-nebulized beclomethasone
        (a) Budesonide (Pulmicort Respules®)
        (b) Flunisolide (AeroBid-M®, AeroBid®)
        (c) Fluticasone (Flovent®)
        (d) Mometasone (Asmanex®)
        (e) Triamcinolone (Azmacort®)
     (3) Systemic
        (a) Dexamethasone
        (b) Prednisone (Deltasone®)
        (c) Methylprednisolone (Medrol®)
   d) Opiates ($$–$$$)—Morphine used orally (immediate release), subcutaneously, parenterally, or sublingually. The effectiveness of extended-release morphine for the management of dyspnea has not been well established.
   e) Anxiolytics (if anxiety present) ($–$$)
     (1) Benzodiazepines
     (2) Phenothiazines
   f) Blood transfusion ($$$) for treatment of anemia
   g) Erythropoietin ($$$) for restoration of red blood cell count and treatment of anemia
   h) Radiation therapy or chemotherapy ($$$) as required to treat disease
  2. **Level II—moderate level of evidence**
   (Bredin et al., 1999; Corner, Plant, A'Hern, & Bailey, 1996; Filshie, Penn, Ashley, & Davis, 1996)
   a) Cognitive-behavioral modifications ($$)
   b) Acupuncture ($$)

B. Death is imminent.
  1. **Level I—high level of evidence**
   (Jennings et al., 2002; Navigante, Cerchietti, Castro, Lutteral, & Cabalar, 2006; Wickham, 1998)
   a) Morphine ($–$$$)—(See previous description.)
   b) Midazolam plus morphine—One well-done randomized trial; more are required to verify.
   c) Anticholinergics ($)—scopolamine, atropine
   d) Terminal sedation if needed (See Palliative Sedation.)
  2. **Level II—moderate level of evidence**
   (Ahmedzai, Laude, Robertson, Troy, & Vora, 2004; Bruera et al., 2003, 2005; Coyne, Viswanathan, & Smith, 2002; Davis, 1999; Jantarakupt & Porock, 2005; Kohara et al., 2003; Quigley, Joel, Patel, Baksh, & Slevin, 2002; Shimoyama & Shimoyama, 2002; Tanaka et al., 1999; Wickham, 1998)
   a) Supplemental oxygen—Use a nasal cannula if possible to improve patient comfort. Because of inconclusive data, oxygen therapy should be

considered on a case-by-case basis with the goal of making the patient as comfortable as possible.

   b) Nebulized fentanyl ($$)

   c) Nebulized furosemide ($)

   d) Nebulized morphine ($)

   e) Acupuncture ($$)

   f) Cognitive-behavioral approaches ($)

Patient Outcomes

A. Dyspnea is minimized.

B. Patient is able to perform activities that are of importance and contribute to quality of life.

C. Patient is able to breathe without discomfort.

References

Ahmedzai, S.H., Laude, E., Robertson, A., Troy, G., & Vora, V. (2004). A double blind, randomized, controlled phase II trial of heliox 28 gas mixture in lung cancer patients with dyspnoea on exertion. *British Journal of Cancer, 90,* 366–371.

Allard, P., Lamontagne, C., Bernard, P., & Tremblay, C. (1999). How effective are supplementary doses of opioids for dyspnea in terminally ill cancer patients? A randomized continuous sequential clinical trial. *Journal of Pain and Symptom Management, 17,* 256–265.

American Thoracic Society. (1999). Dyspnea mechanisms, assessment and management: A consensus statement. *American Journal of Respiratory and Critical Care Medicine, 159,* 321–340.

Bredin, M., Corner, J., Krishnasamy, M., Plant, H., Bailey, C., & A'Hern, R. (1999). Multicenter randomized controlled trial of nursing intervention for breathlessness in patients with lung cancer. *BMJ, 318,* 901–904.

Bruera, E., Macmillan, K., Pither, J., & MacDonald, R.N. (1990). Effects of morphine on the dyspnea of terminal cancer patients. *Journal of Pain and Symptom Management, 5,* 341–344.

Bruera, E., Sala, R., Spruyt, O., Palmer, J.L., Zhang, T., & Willey, J. (2005). Nebulized versus subcutaneous morphine for patients with cancer dyspnea: A preliminary study. *Journal of Pain and Symptom Management, 29,* 613–618.

Bruera, E., Sweeney, C., Willey, J., Palmer, J.L., Strasser, F., & Morice, R.C. (2003). Randomized controlled trial of supplemental oxygen versus air in cancer patients with dyspnea. *Palliative Medicine, 17,* 659–663.

Corner, J., Plant, H., A'Hern, R., & Bailey, C. (1996). Non-pharmacological intervention for breathlessness in lung cancer. *Palliative Medicine, 10,* 299–305.

Coyne, P.J., Viswanathan, R., & Smith, T.J. (2002). Nebulized fentanyl citrate improves patients' perception of breathing, respiratory rate, and oxygen saturation in dyspnea. *Journal of Pain and Symptom Management, 23,* 157–160.

Davis, C. (1999). Palliation of breathlessness. In C. von Gunten (Ed.), *Palliative care and rehabilitation of cancer patients* (pp. 59–74). Boston: Kluwer Academic.

Dudgeon, D. (2005). Management of dyspnea at the end of life. In D. Mahler & D. O'Donnell (Eds.), *Dyspnea: Mechanisms, measurement and management* (2nd ed., pp. 429–461). Boca Raton, FL: Taylor & Francis.

Filshie, J., Penn, K., Ashley, S., & Davis, C.L. (1996). Acupuncture for the relief of cancer-related breathlessness. *Palliative Medicine, 10,* 145–150.

Jantarakupt, P., & Porock, D. (2005). Dyspnea management in lung cancer: Applying the evidence from chronic obstructive pulmonary disease. *Oncology Nursing Forum, 32,* 785–795.

Jennings, A., Davies, A., Higgins, P., Gibbs, J., & Broadley, K. (2002). A systematic review of the use of opioids in the management of dyspnea. *Thorax, 57,* 939–944.

Joyce, M., McSweeney, M., Carrieri-Kohlman, V.L., & Hawkins, J. (2004). The use of nebulized opioids in the management of dyspnea: Evidence synthesis. *Oncology Nursing Forum, 31,* 551–561.

Kohara, H., Ueoka, H., Aoe, K., Maeda, T., Takeyama, H., Saito, R., et al. (2003). Effect of nebulized furosemide in terminally ill cancer patients with dyspnea. *Journal of Pain and Symptom Management, 26,* 962–967.

Kuebler, K.K., Andry, J.M., & Davis, S. (2007). Dyspnea. In K.K. Kuebler, D.E. Heidrich, & P. Esper (Eds.), *Palliative and end-of-life care: Clinical practice guidelines* (2nd ed., pp. 377–394). St. Louis, MO: Elsevier Saunders.

Mazzocato, C., Buclin, T., & Rapin, C.H. (1999). The effects of morphine on dyspnea and ventilatory function in elderly patients with advanced cancer: A randomized double-blind controlled trial. *Annals of Oncology, 10,* 1511–1514.

Navigante, A.H., Cerchietti, L.C., Castro, M.A., Lutteral, M.A., & Cabalar, M.E. (2006). Midazolam as adjunct therapy to morphine in the alleviation of severe dyspnea perception in patients with advanced cancer. *Journal of Pain and Symptom Management, 31,* 38–47.

Pereira, J., & Bruera, E. (1997). *The Edmonton aid to palliative care.* Edmonton, Canada: Division of Palliative Care, University of Alberta.

Quigley, C., Joel, S., Patel, N., Baksh, A., & Slevin, M. (2002). A phase I/II study of nebulized morphine-6-glucuronide in patients with cancer-related breathlessness. *Journal of Pain and Symptom Management, 23,* 7–9.

Rao, A., & Gray, D. (2003). Breathlessness in hospitalized adult patients. *Postgraduate Medical Journal, 79,* 681–685.

Sharp, J., Drutz, W., Moisan, T., Foster, J., & Machnach, W. (1980). Postural relief of dyspnea in severe chronic pulmonary disease. *American Review of Respiratory Disease, 122,* 201–211.

Shimoyama, N., & Shimoyama, M. (2002). Nebulized furosemide as a novel treatment for dyspnea in terminal cancer patients. *Journal of Pain and Symptom Management, 23,* 73–76.

Tanaka, K., Shima, Y., Kakinuma, R., Kubota, K., Ohe, Y., & Hojo, F. (1999). Effect of nebulized morphine in cancer patients with dyspnea: A pilot study. *Japanese Journal of Clinical Oncology, 29,* 600–603.

Thomas, J., & von Gunten, C. (2003). Management of dyspnea. *Journal of Supportive Oncology, 1,* 23–34.

Waller, A., & Caroline N. (2000). *Handbook of palliative care in cancer* (2nd ed.). Woburn, MA: Butterworth-Heinemann.

Wickham, R. (1998). Managing dyspnea in cancer patients. *Development in Supportive Cancer Care, 2*(2), 33–40.

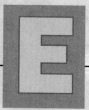

Edema

Edema

Debra E. Heidrich, MSN, RN, ACHPN®, AOCN®

Definition

Edema is the abnormal accumulation of fluid in the intracellular spaces.

Pathophysiology and Etiology

Edema is the result of a number of pathophysiologic alterations that lead to either fluid overload or failure to excrete fluids (White, 2005). In palliative care, common causes of edema are cardiac, renal, or hepatic failure; hypoalbuminemia; syndrome of inappropriate antidiuretic hormone secretion (SIADH); and immobility. (Small cell lung cancer is the most common cause of SIADH.) Administration of enteral or parenteral fluids in the presence of renal or cardiac compromise will lead to edema. Medications, such as corticosteroids and some hormonal agents, will contribute to edema. Edema interferes with the normal exchange of nutrition and excretion within cells, leading to an increased risk of tissue breakdown (Waller & Caroline, 2000; White).

Manifestations

- Swollen extremities with or without pitting
- Pale and cool skin
- Discomfort in edematous tissue
- Tissue breakdown
- Weeping of skin
- Dyspnea

With SIADH, the following symptoms are seen.
- Fatigue or lethargy
- Muscle cramps
- Nausea and vomiting
- Headache
- Severe confusion, seizures, or coma

Management

A. Death is not imminent.
   1. Pharmacologic interventions
      a) **Level I—high level of evidence**
      Diuretics are helpful for fluid overload associated with heart failure, but carefully evaluate benefits and burdens.
      (1) Furosemide (Lasix®) ($) 20–40 mg po daily or spironolactone (Aldactone®) ($$) 100 mg po daily may be helpful. Dosages may be increased if not effective after several days.
      (2) Administer diuretics in the morning.
      (3) Evaluate the patient's ability to reach the bathroom or a bedside commode quickly and the energy expenditure that this requires. Catheterization of the bladder may be necessary to promote comfort and save energy for other activities valued by the patient.
      (4) Monitor for hypotension, hypokalemia, and hyponatremia.
      b) **Level II—moderate level of evidence**
      (1) Use demeclocycline (Declomycin®) ($$$) to treat SIADH—300 mg po bid interferes with the antidiuretic hormone effect on renal tubules and promotes fluid excretion by the kidneys (Bower & Cox, 2004; Twycross & Wilcock, 2006).
      (2) IV infusion of 0.9%–3% saline, in combination with diuretics ($$$), is reserved for severe hyponatremia, when the patient's functional status is likely to improve with treatment (Bower & Cox, 2004; Waller & Caroline, 2000). If functional status is not likely to improve, this intervention should not be used in the palliative care setting.
   2. Nonpharmacologic interventions
      Level III—low level of evidence
      These interventions are widely accepted as beneficial, but little evidence-based research is available in this area.
      a) Encourage exercise, as tolerated, to improve circulation. Walking, active or passive range of motion, and isometric exercises are helpful (Waller & Caroline, 2000).
      b) Encourage use of compression stockings ($$) if the patient is active. Bedridden patients do not benefit by using compression stockings (Waller & Caroline, 2000).
      c) Elevate edematous extremities to the level of the heart or above.
      d) Dietary changes are rarely helpful in the palliative care setting. If the patient feels like eating, encourage high-protein foods. Fluid and sodium restrictions are not appropriate.
      e) Restriction of free fluid intake to < 500 ml/day generally is considered helpful (Bower & Cox, 2004) but is considered burdensome in the palliative care setting (Twycross & Wilcock, 2006).
      f) Decrease or discontinue enteral or parenteral fluids if they are contributing to edema.

g) Protect skin with moisturizers, gentle handling, and appropriate positioning and support to minimize pressure.

B. Death is imminent.
  1. Continue to provide excellent skin care.
  2. Elevate edematous extremities if this promotes comfort.
  3. Discontinue diuretics unless the patient is catheterized. As death approaches, assess for the need to continue diuretics.
  4. Discontinue enteral or parenteral fluids if they are causing edema.

Patient Outcomes

A. Comfort is maintained.

B. Functional status is optimal.

C. Patient is free of any symptoms of skin breakdown.

References

Bower, M., & Cox, S. (2004). Endocrine and metabolic complications of advanced cancer. In D. Doyle, G. Hanks, N. Cherny, & K. Calman (Eds.), *Oxford textbook of palliative medicine* (3rd ed., pp. 687–702). New York: Oxford University Press.

Twycross, R., & Wilcock, A. (Eds.). (2006). *Hospice and palliative care formulary USA*. Nottingham, UK: Palliativedrugs.com Ltd.

Waller, A., & Caroline, N.L. (2000). *Handbook of palliative care in cancer*. Boston: Butterworth-Heinemann.

White, B. (2005). Clients with fluid imbalances. In J.M. Black & J.H. Hawks (Eds.), *Medical-surgical nursing: Clinical management for positive outcomes* (7th ed., pp. 205–221). St. Louis, MO: Elsevier Saunders.

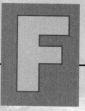

Fatigue

Fever

Funeral Planning

Fatigue

Jennifer Fournier, RN, MSN, AOCN®, CHPN

Definition

Fatigue has been recently redefined as an adaptive state along a continuum be-tween tiredness and exhaustion (Olson, 2007). The palliative care patient experiences multifaceted and complex fatigue that tends to be undertreated and underdiagnosed. Fatigue is a subjective sensation and may be the most distressing symptom to the palliative care patient (Hofman, Ryan, Figueroa-Moseley, Jean-Pierre, & Morrow, 2007). In fatigue, the degree of energy depletion is not correlated to energy used, and the affected individual must make a conscious effort to perform priority tasks. Heightened anxiety, confusion, decreased physical functioning, depression, and a lower quality of life may be present in fatigued patients (Barnes et al., 2006; Burst-ein, 2007; Fernandes, Stone, Andrews, Morgan, & Sharma, 2006; Kim, Hickok, & Morrow, 2006; Morrow, 2007; Tsai et al., 2007).

Pathophysiology and Etiology

Fatigue may be influenced by a variety of physiologic and psychological compo-nents, and it is the most common symptom seen in the last year of life (Doorenbos, Given, Given, & Verbitsky, 2006). Fifteen percent to 91% of patients experience some level of fatigue (Barnes et al., 2006; Berger, Farr, Kuhn, Fischer, & Agrawal, 2007; Ferreri, Agbokou, & Gauthier, 2006; Hacker & Ferrans, 2007; Henry, Viswa-nathan, Wade, Servin, & Cella, 2006; Hofman et al., 2007; McMillan, Dunbar, & Zhang, 2007; Piche et al., 2005; So & Tai, 2005; Yurtsever, 2007). Conflicting evidence exists regarding the role of gender in predicting the occurrence of fatigue (Husain et al., 2007; Kim et al., 2006; Yurtsever).

Sleep disturbance, vomiting, nausea, constipation, infection, anorexia, anemia, metabolic imbalance, and dyspnea have been linked to fatigue (Fernandes et al., 2006; Hofman et al., 2007; Morrow, Shelke, Roscoe, Hickok, & Mustian, 2005; Roscoe et al., 2007; Tsai et al., 2007). Treatments for cancer (radiation, biotherapy,

The author would like to acknowledge Beth Cohen, RNC, ARNP, MSN, for her contribution that remains unchanged from the first edition of this textbook.

and chemotherapy) can result in increased fatigue for months to years (Morrow, 2007; So & Tai, 2005; Thompson, 2007), which may result in more detrimental complications for older patients (Balducci, 2007; Morrow). Palliative care patients also may experience fatigue related to medication side effects, tests, procedures, or chronic pain. Additionally, emotional distress of anxiety or depression may contribute to increased fatigue (National Comprehensive Cancer Network [NCCN], 2007).

The release of pro-inflammatory cytokines during cancer treatment may precipitate fatigue (Ganz, 2006; Morrow, 2007; Morrow et al., 2005; Rich, 2007; Ryan et al., 2007). Additionally, a theory exists that the disruption of the circadian rhythm by targeted signaling from epidermal growth factor receptors (EGFRs) by either a tumor or the host in patients with cancer may lead to increased fatigue (Rich). Another possible cause of fatigue may involve the dysregulation of brain serotonin (5-HT) levels (Ryan et al.). The use of the 5-HT_3 receptor antagonist ondansetron has shown promising results in the treatment of fatigue related to chronic hepatitis C (Piche et al., 2005).

Manifestations
- Sleep disturbances
- Feeling cold
- Weakness
- Tiredness
- Anxiety
- Forgetfulness
- Increased sensitivity to stimuli
- Weariness
- Apprehension
- Nausea
- Impaired socialization
- Lassitude
- Inattention
- Diarrhea

Management
A. General measures
   1. Assess for cause and treat as appropriate.
   2. Some causes include pulmonary, renal, cardiac, hepatic, or neurologic dysfunctions; anemia; hypothyroidism; infection; insomnia; pain; malnutrition; and emotional distress.

B. Death is not imminent.
   1. **Level I—high level of evidence**
      (Berger, Kallich, & Oster, 2006; Burstein, 2007; Carroll, Kohli, Mustian, Roscoe, & Morrow, 2007; Cassileth, 2006; Chen et al., 2006; DeBattista,

Doghramji, Menza, Rosenthal, & Fieve, 2003; Gale, 2006; Henry, Williams, Xie, & Willhelm, 2007; Kurtin, 2007; Meyer, 2007; Mitchell, Beck, Hood, Moore, & Tanner, 2007; Morrow, 2007; Morrow et al., 2005; Mustian et al., 2007; NCCN, 2007; Oestreicher, 2007; Oken et al., 2006; Penninx, Cohen, & Woodman, 2007; Piche et al., 2005; Ross et al., 2006; Schartzberg et al., 2006; Smith, 2007; So & Tai, 2005; *Tarascon Pocket Pharmacopoeia,* 2004; U.S. Food and Drug Administration, 2007a, 2007b; Vandebroek et al., 2006)

a) Exercise

b) Erythropoiesis-stimulating agents (ESAs) (only for chemotherapy-induced anemia)

    (1) For anemia, balance benefit with potential harm; target hemoglobin level of 10 g/dl

    (2) Epoetin alfa (Procrit®, Epogen®) ($$$)—40,000 units subcutaneously (SC) weekly or 80,000 units SC every two weeks

    (3) Darbepoetin alfa (Aranesp®) ($$$)—200–500 mcg SC every one to four weeks

c) Psychostimulant

    (1) Modafinil (Provigil®) ($$$)—100–400 mg po one to two times daily

    (2) Lower doses may be more effective; significantly decreased abuse potential; generally well tolerated

2. **Level II—moderate level of evidence**
(Carroll et al., 2007; Meyer, 2007; Mitchell et al., 2007; Morrow, 2007; Morrow et al., 2005; Mustian, 2007; NCCN, 2007; *Tarascon Pocket Pharmacopoeia,* 2004)

a) Psychostimulants

    (1) Methylphenidate (Ritalin®) ($)—5–50 mg po daily

    (2) Dexmethylphenidate (Focalin®) ($$)—2.5 mg po bid, titrate; maximum 20 mg/day

    (3) Dextroamphetamine (Dexedrine®) ($$)—2.5–10 mg po one to three times daily

b) Donepezil (Aricept®) ($$$)—5 mg every morning (may have dose-limiting side effects)

c) Bupropion sustained-release (Wellbutrin SR®) ($$$)—100–150 mg po daily

d) Psychotherapy and cognitive therapy

e) Complementary therapies

    (1) Acupuncture

    (2) Polarity therapy, an energy therapy using gentle touch to balance an individual's energy field to restore health

f) Low-dose corticosteroids

    (1) Prednisone ($)—5–10 mg po daily

    (2) Dexamethasone ($)—1–2 mg po bid

3. **Level III—low level of evidence**

(Bardia, Greeno, & Bauer, 2007; Cassileth, 2006; Mitchell et al., 2007; NCCN, 2007; Oestreicher, 2007; Oncology Nursing Society, n.d.)
   a) Massage
   b) Energy preservation
   c) Progressive muscle relaxation
   d) Sleep therapy
   e) Healing touch (an energy therapy used to balance an individual's energy field that does not use actual physical contact)
   f) Yoga
   g) Supplements (may cause drug interactions)
      (1) Chondroitin
      (2) Shark cartilage
      (3) Echinacea
      (4) Ginkgo
      (5) Ginseng
      (6) Ginger
      (7) Mistletoe
      (8) Garlic
      (9) Green tea
      (10) Iron
   h) Stress management
   i) Prayer
   j) Adequate nutrition and hydration
   k) Relaxation

C. Death is imminent.
   1. Treatment of fatigue should be discontinued as death approaches.
   2. Comfort measures should be continued or initiated as appropriate.

Patient Outcomes

A. Fatigue is relieved or decreased to an acceptable level.

B. Patient comfort is maintained.

C. Patient has sufficient energy to perform important tasks.

References

Balducci, L. (2007). An overlooked problem: Anemia in the elderly patient with cancer. *Journal of Supportive Oncology, 5,* 115–116.

Bardia, A., Greeno, E., & Bauer, B.A. (2007). Dietary supplement usage by patients with cancer undergoing chemotherapy: Does prognosis or cancer symptoms predict usage? *Journal of Supportive Oncology, 5,* 195–198.

Barnes, S., Gott, M., Payne, S., Parker, C., Seamark, D., Gariballa, S., et al. (2006). Prevalence of symptoms in a community-based sample of heart failure patients. *Journal of Pain and Symptom Management, 32,* 208–216.

Berger, A.M., Farr, L.A., Kuhn, B.R., Fischer, P., & Agrawal, S. (2007). Values of sleep/wake, activity/ rest, circadian rhythms, and fatigue prior to adjuvant breast cancer chemotherapy. *Journal of Pain and Symptom Management, 33,* 398–409.

Berger, A., Kallich, J., & Oster, G. (2006, June). *Use of darbepoetin alfa and epoetin alfa for anemia in clinical practice.* Paper presented at the 18th Annual Symposium of the Multinational Association of Supportive Care in Cancer, Toronto, Canada.

Burstein, H.J. (2007). Anemia in cancer: Update on studies of erythropoiesis-stimulating agents. *Journal of Supportive Oncology, 5*(Suppl. 2), 5–7.

Carroll, J.K., Kohli, S., Mustian, K.M., Roscoe, J.A., & Morrow, G.R. (2007). Pharmacologic treatment of cancer-related fatigue. *Oncologist, 12*(Suppl.1), 43–51.

Cassileth, B.R. (2006, September). *Integrative oncology: Complementary therapy for cancer survivors.* Paper presented at the Second Annual Chicago Supportive Oncology Conference, Chicago, IL.

Chen, E., Peake, C., Buscaino, E., Forlenza, J., Bookhart, B., & McKenzie, R.S. (2006, December). *Hematologic outcomes and erythropoiesis-stimulating therapy costs in epoetin alfa- and darbepoetin alfa-treated cancer patients: Results of the dosing and outcomes study of erythropoiesis-stimulating therapies (DOSE) registry* [Abstract 3340]. Paper presented at the 48th annual meeting of the American Society of Hematology, Orlando, FL.

DeBattista, C., Doghramji, K., Menza, M.A., Rosenthal, M.H., & Fieve, R.R. (2003). Adjunct modafinil for the short-term treatment of fatigue and sleepiness in patients with major depressive disorder: A preliminary double-blind, placebo-controlled study. *Journal of Clinical Psychiatry, 64,* 1057–1064.

Doorenbos, A.Z., Given, C.W., Given, B., & Verbitsky, N. (2006). Symptom experience in the last year of life among individuals with cancer. *Journal of Pain and Symptom Management, 32,* 403–412.

Fernandes, R., Stone, P., Andrews, P., Morgan, R., & Sharma, S. (2006). Comparison between fatigue, sleep disturbance, and circadian rhythm in cancer inpatients and healthy volunteers: Evaluation of diagnostic criteria for cancer-related fatigue. *Journal of Pain and Symptom Management, 32,* 245–254.

Ferreri, F., Agbokou, C., & Gauthier, S. (2006). Recognition and management of neuropsychiatric complications in Parkinson's disease. *Canadian Medical Association Journal, 175,* 1545–1552.

Gale, K. (2006, May 22). *Modafinil reduces fatigue in patients with fibromyalgia.* Retrieved May 15, 2007, from http://www.medscape.com/viewarticle/532948

Ganz, P. (2006, September). *Cancer survivors: Issues in symptom management.* Paper presented at the Second Annual Chicago Supportive Oncology Conference, Chicago, IL.

Hacker, E.D., & Ferrans, C.E. (2007). Ecological momentary assessment of fatigue in patients receiving intensive cancer therapy. *Journal of Pain and Symptom Management, 33,* 267–275.

Henry, D.H., Viswanathan, H.N., Wade, S.M., Servin, M., & Cella, D. (2006, December). *The patient's experience of fatigue: A cross-sectional study of cancer* [Abstract 3356]. Paper presented at the 48th annual meeting of the American Society of Hematology, Orlando, FL.

Henry, D.H., Williams, D., Xie, J., & Wilhelm, F. (2007). Randomized, open-label comparison of epoetin alfa extended dosing (80,000 U every two weeks) versus weekly dosing (40,000 U weekly) in anemic patients with cancer receiving chemotherapy [Abstract]. *Journal of Supportive Oncology, 5*(Suppl. 2), 17.

Hofman, M., Ryan, J.L., Figueroa-Moseley, C.D., Jean-Pierre, P., & Morrow, G.R. (2007). Cancer-related fatigue: The scale of the problem. *Oncologist, 12*(Suppl. 1), 4–10.

Husain, A.F., Stewart, K., Arseneault, R., Moineddin, R., Cellarius, V., Librach, L., et al. (2007). Women experience higher levels of fatigue than men at the end of life: A longitudinal home palliative care study. *Journal of Pain and Symptom Management, 33,* 389–397.

Kim, Y., Hickok, J.T., & Morrow, G. (2006). Fatigue and depression in cancer patients undergoing chemotherapy: An emotion approach. *Journal of Pain and Symptom Management, 32,* 311–321.

Kurtin, S.E. (2007). A time for hope: Promising advances in the management of anemia, neutropenia, thrombocytopenia, and mucositis. *Journal of Supportive Oncology, 5*(Suppl. 2), 85–88.

McMillan, S.C., Dunbar, S.B., & Zhang, W. (2007). The prevalence of symptoms in hospice patients with end-stage heart disease. *Journal of Hospice and Palliative Nursing, 9,* 124–131.

Meyer, L.P. (2007). Fatigue. In K.K. Kuebler, D.E. Heidrich, & P. Esper (Eds.), *Palliative and end-of-life care: Clinical practice guidelines* (2nd ed., pp. 395–409). St. Louis, MO: Elsevier Saunders.

Mitchell, S.A., Beck, S.L., Hood, L.E., Moore, K., & Tanner, E.R. (2007). Putting evidence into practice: Evidence-based interventions for fatigue during and following cancer and its treatment. *Clinical Journal of Oncology Nursing, 11,* 99–113.

Morrow, G.R. (2007). Cancer-related fatigue: Causes, consequences, and management. *Oncologist, 12*(Suppl. 1), 1–3.

Morrow, G.R., Shelke, A.R., Roscoe, J.A., Hickok, J.T., & Mustian, K. (2005). Management of cancer-related fatigue. *Cancer Investigation, 23,* 229–239.

Mustian, K.M., Morrow, G.R., Carroll, J.K., Figueroa-Moseley, C.D., Jean-Pierre, P., & Williams, G.C. (2007). Integrative nonpharmacologic behavioral interventions for the management of cancer-related fatigue. *Oncologist, 12*(Suppl. 1), 52–67.

National Comprehensive Cancer Network. (2007, April). *NCCN clinical practice guidelines in oncology: Cancer-related fatigue, version 3.2007.* Retrieved April 29, 2007, from http://www.nccn.org/professionals/physician_gls/PDF/fatigue.pdf

Oestreicher, P. (2007, March). What nursing interventions improve fatigue in patients with cancer? *ONS Connect, 22*(3), 22–23.

Oken, B.S., Zajdel, D., Kishiyama, S., Flegal, K., Dehen, C., Haas, M., et al. (2006). Randomized, controlled, six-month trial of yoga in healthy seniors: Effects on cognition and quality of life. *Alternative Therapies, 12,* 40–47.

Olson, K. (2007). A new way of thinking about fatigue: A reconceptualization. *Oncology Nursing Forum, 34,* 93–99.

Oncology Nursing Society. (n.d.). *Measuring oncology nursing-sensitive patient outcomes: Evidence-based summary.* Retrieved May 1, 2007, from http://www.ons.org/outcomes/measures/pdfFatigueSummary.pdf

Penninx, B.W., Cohen, H.J., & Woodman, R.C. (2007). Anemia and cancer in older persons. *Journal of Supportive Oncology, 5,* 107–113.

Piche, T., Vanbiervliet, G., Cherikh, F., Antoun, Z., Huet, P.M., Gelsi, E., et al. (2005). Effect of ondansetron, a 5-HT3 receptor antagonist, on fatigue in chronic hepatitis C: A randomized, double blind, placebo controlled study. *Gut, 54,* 1169–1173.

Rich, T.A. (2007). Symptom clusters in cancer patients and their relation to EGFR ligand modulation of the circadian axis. *Journal of Supportive Oncology, 5,* 167–174.

Roscoe, J.A., Kaufman, M.E., Matteson-Rusby, S.E., Palesh, O.G., Ryan, J.L., Kohli, S., et al. (2007). Cancer-related fatigue and sleep disorders. *Oncologist, 12*(Suppl. 1), 35–42.

Ross, S.D., Allen, I.E., Henry, D., Seaman, C., Sercus, B., & Goodnough, L.T. (2006, June). *Clinical benefits and risks associated with epoetin (alfa/beta) and darbepoetin alfa in patients with chemotherapy-induced anemia: A systematic review of the literature* [Abstract 02-006]. Paper presented at the 18th Annual Symposium of the Multinational Association of Supportive Care in Cancer, Toronto, Canada.

Ryan, J.L., Carroll, J.K., Ryan, E.P., Mustian, K.M., Fiscella, K., & Morrow, G.R. (2007). Mechanisms of cancer-related fatigue. *Oncologist, 12*(Suppl. 1), 22–34.

Schwartzberg, L., Rearden, T., Yee, L., Mirtsching, B., Charu, V., Lam, H., et al. (2006, December). *A phase II, randomized, open-label study to assess the efficacy of extended-dose schedule administration of darbepoetin alfa in cancer patients with chemotherapy-induced anemia* [Abstract 1306]. Paper presented at the 48th annual meeting of the American Society of Hematology, Orlando, FL.

Smith, J.A. (2007). Implementation of cytokines to optimize cancer treatment outcomes. *Journal of Supportive Oncology, 5*(Suppl. 2), 89–91.

So, W.K., & Tai, J.W. (2005). Fatigue and fatigue-relieving strategies used by Hong Kong Chinese patients after hemopoietic stem cell transplantation. *Nursing Research, 54,* 48–55.

Tarascon pocket pharmacopoeia (2004 classic shirt-pocket ed.). (2004). Lompoc, CA: Tarascon.

Thompson, P. (2007). The relationship of fatigue and meaning of life in breast cancer survivors. *Oncology Nursing Forum, 34,* 653–660.

Tsai, L., Li, I., Lai, Y., Liu, C., Chang, T., & Tu, C. (2007). Fatigue and its associated factors in hospice cancer patients in Taiwan. *Cancer Nursing, 30,* 24–30.

U.S. Food and Drug Administration. (2007a, November 8). FDA public health advisory: Erythropoiesis-stimulating agents (ESAS): *Epoetin alfa (marketed as Procrit, Epogen), darbepoetin (marketed as Aranesp).* Retrieved April 29, 2007, from http://www.fda.gov/cder/drug/advisory/RHE200711.htm

U.S. Food and Drug Administration. (2007b, November 8). *Information for healthcare professionals: Erythropoiesis stimulating agents (ESA) [Aranesp (darbepoetin), Epogen (epoetin alfa), and Procrit (epoetin alfa)].* Retrieved April 29, 2007, from http://www.fda.gov/cder/drug/InfoSheets/HCP/RHE200711HCP.htm

Vandebroek, A., Gaede, B., Altintas, S., Smith, K., Yao, B., Schupp, M., et al. (2006, June). *A randomized open-label study of darbepoetin alfa administered every 3 weeks with or without parenteral iron in anemic subjects with nonmyeloid malignancies receiving chemotherapy* [Abstract 8612]. Paper presented at the 42nd annual meeting of the American Society of Clinical Oncology, Atlanta, GA.

Yurtsever, S. (2007). The experience of fatigue in Turkish patients receiving chemotherapy. *Oncology Nursing Forum, 34,* 721–728.

Fever

John Travis Dunlap, MSN, ANP-BC, and George E. Holburn, MSN

Definition

Fever is a state characterized by an elevation of core body temperature occurring in response to pyrogens.

Pathophysiology and Etiology

The normal body temperature "set point" is regulated by the hypothalamus and varies from person to person and the time of day (e.g., circadian rhythm). Several studies demonstrated that lower temperatures typically occur around dawn, and higher temperatures are seen in the late afternoon (Yoon et al., 2003). Fever not only occurs in response to an infectious process but also is present in the inflammatory processes, such as trauma, surgery, or burns, as well as in an autoimmune response, such as rheumatoid arthritis or malignant tumors. Patients who are actively dying often experience a febrile state (Hall, Schroder, & Weaver, 2002).

Manifestations

- Fatigue
- Skin warmth
- Tachycardia
- Dizziness
- Shortness of breath
- Diaphoresis
- Cold intolerance
- Flushed cheeks
- Headache
- Decreased appetite (anorexia)
- Delirium
- Weakness

The authors would like to acknowledge Beth Cohen, RNC, ARNP, MSN, for her contribution that remains unchanged from the first edition of this textbook.

- Chills
- Body aches
- Lethargy

(Blum, 2006)

Management

A. Death is not imminent.
   1. **Level I—high level of evidence**
      a) Antipyretic medications
         (1) Acetaminophen ($)
           (a) Acetaminophen is available as a tablet, a chewable tablet, a capsule, a suspension or solution (liquid), drops (concentrated liquid), an extended-release (long-acting) tablet, and an orally disintegrating tablet (tablet that dissolves quickly in the mouth), to take by mouth with or without food. Acetaminophen also is available as a suppository to use rectally (pr).
           (b) Adults—500–1,000 mg every four to six hours po or pr. Do not exceed 4 g/day (Munir, Enany, & Zhang, 2007).
         (2) Ibuprofen ($)
           (a) Ibuprofen is available in a tablet form to take by mouth, usually three or four times a day for arthritis or every four to six hours as needed for pain (Munir et al., 2007). Nonprescription ibuprofen can be formed as a tablet, a chewable tablet, a suspension (liquid), and drops (concentrated liquid).
           (b) Adults—200–400 mg every four to six hours po. Do not exceed 2,400 mg/day (Munir et al., 2007).
         (3) Aspirin ($)
           (a) Prescription aspirin is an extended-release tablet (a tablet that releases medication slowly over a period of time). Nonprescription aspirin is available in a tablet, an enteric-coated tablet, or a delayed-release tablet (a tablet that begins to release medication some time after it is taken), a chewable tablet, and a gum or as a suppository for rectal administration.
           (b) Adults—500–1,000 mg every four to six hours po or pr. Do not exceed 4 g/day (Munir et al., 2007).
           (c) The side effects vary with the specific medication ordered and include abdominal discomfort, heartburn, tinnitus, and liver function alterations.
           (d) If the patient is on oral pain relievers that combine two or more drugs, including an antipyretic, care must be taken not to exceed the total daily dose of antipyretic medication allowed.
           (e) Suppository use is contraindicated in patients with bowel obstruction, diarrhea, and problematic hemorrhoids and in patients receiving chemotherapy who are neutropenic.

(f) Enteric-coated pills should never be crushed prior to adminis-tration (Hodgson & Kizior, 2007).

(4) Hydration ($–$$)

(a) Encourage the patient to drink fluids when able, especially to replace fluids in the setting of vomiting and diarrhea.

(b) Urine output (the patient should have several wet diapers or frequent trips to the bathroom daily), saliva in the mouth, and moist eyes are important assessment parameters when evaluating dehydration (Kedziera & Coyle, 2006). (See Dehydration.)

(5) Antibiotics ($$–$$$)

(a) Antibiotic use should be considered if an infection is present.

(b) Antibiotic use should be based upon sensitivities derived from culture results.

(c) Administration may be po or IV (Chen et al., 2002; Hodgson & Kizior, 2007; Holtzclaw, 2003).

2. **Level III—low level of evidence**

Comfort measures

a) Do not bundle a patient who has the chills.

b) Remove excess clothing or blankets. The environment should be comfortably cool. For example, consider one layer of lightweight clothing with one lightweight blanket to sleep. If the room is hot or stuffy, using a fan or opening a window may be helpful.

c) A lukewarm bath or sponge bath may help to cool someone with a fever, which is especially effective after an antipyretic is given; otherwise, the temperature may quickly rebound.

d) Do not use cold baths or alcohol rubs, which cool the skin but often make the situation worse by causing shivering that raises the core body temperature.

e) Encourage the patient to drink cool liquids, as tolerated (Medline Plus, 2006).

B. Death is imminent.

1. Comfort measures should continue.

2. Treating the cause of the fever may be abandoned, depending on the wishes of the patient and family.

3. Supportive comfort care should be emphasized in the patient who is dying, and the use of antipyretic and hydration therapies should be considered in individual patient situations.

Patient Outcomes

A. Fever is reduced or prevented.

B. Comfort is increased.

C. Anxiety is reduced for the patient and caregivers.

References

Blum, F.C. (2006). Fever in the adult patient. In J.A. Marx, R.S. Hockberger, & R.M. Walls (Eds.), *Rosen's emergency medicine: Concepts and clinical practice* (6th ed., pp. 134–137). St. Louis, MO: Mosby.

Chen, L.K., Chou, Y.C., Hsu, P.S., Tsai, S.T., Hwang, S.J., Wu, B.Y., et al. (2002). Antibiotic prescription for fever episodes in hospice patients. *Supportive Care in Cancer, 10,* 538–541.

Hall, P., Schroder, C., & Weaver, L. (2002). The last 48 hours of life in long-term care: A focused chart audit. *Journal of the American Geriatrics Society, 50,* 501–506.

Hodgson, B., & Kizior, R. (2007). *Saunders nursing drug handbook 2008.* St. Louis, MO: Elsevier Saunders.

Holtzclaw, B. (2003). Fever. In C.A. Kirton (Ed.), *ANAC's core curriculum for HIV/AIDS nursing* (2nd ed., pp. 135–137). Thousand Oaks, CA: Sage Publications.

Kedziera, P., & Coyle, N. (2006). Hydration, thirst, and nutrition. In B.R. Ferrell & N. Coyle (Eds.), *Textbook of palliative nursing* (2nd ed., pp. 239–248). New York: Oxford University Press.

Medline Plus. (2006, May 12). *Medline Plus medical encyclopedia—Fever.* Retrieved May 1, 2007, from http://www.nlm.nih.gov/medlineplus/ency/article/003090.htm

Munir, M.A., Enany, N., & Zhang, J.M. (2007). Nonopioid analgesics. *Medical Clinics of North America, 9,* 97–111.

Yoon, I.Y., Kripke, D.F., Elliott, J.A., Youngstedt, S.D., Rex, K.M., & Hauger, R.L. (2003). Age-related changes of circadian rhythms and sleep-wake cycles. *Journal of the American Geriatrics Society, 51,* 1085–1091.

Funeral Planning

Donald Garrison, Lic. Funeral Dir. & Emb.,
Catherine J. Stewart, BSN, RN, APN, Kathryn J. Hill, MSN, BS, MA, APRN, NP-C,
and James C. Pace, DSN, RN, MDiv, ANP-BC, FAANP

Definition

Funeral planning is a process of open communication among the patient, family members, related significant others, healthcare professionals, legal representatives, and funeral home professionals regarding plans for body and property disposition following the patient's death. The planning phase involves spiritual and religious care preparations, financial planning, and wishes regarding body donation and advance directive planning.

Specific Issues in Palliative Care

Background Information

The impact of an aging society will have a burgeoning effect on funeral planning. By 2020, despite advanced and lifesaving technologies in health care, the death rate per 1,000 individuals will approximate the rate in 1960 of nearly 10%, which identifies the need for funeral planning (SmithBucklin Corporation, 2006). Regarding location at time of death, a 1999 study demonstrated that 58% of patients died in hospitals, 22% at home, and 22% in nursing homes; 59% of all hospital deaths occurred in intensive care units (ICUs) (Angus et al., 2004). In reviewing choice of burial, in the 1980s, the rate for cremation (as opposed to full-body burial) reached double digits for the first time and is steadily increasing at an annual rate of 8% (SmithBucklin Corporation). Based on these projections, by 2010, an estimated 36% will choose cremation. Of those cremated in 2005, approximately 90% were Caucasian, 5% were African American, 2% were Asian, and 3% were Hispanic. On average, more men than women choose cremation (54% to 46%, respectively) (SmithBucklin Corporation).

Specific Issues Encountered by Licensed Funeral Home Directors and Families

When death is near, or in cases where arrangements are preplanned, a funeral home director (FHD) meets with the patient and his or her family and friends.

The authors would like to acknowledge Jerre Cory, MA, CSW, for her contribution that remains unchanged from the first edition of this textbook.

Such a meeting ensures that the wishes of the patient and family are clarified and can be realistically and financially accomplished after death. When the patient dies prior to a preplanned meeting, the FHD schedules a meeting with the family at the patient's residence or funeral home. The FHD begins the process of encouraging family members to verbalize the most memorable and honorable details about their loved one.

Most families are not prepared for the amount of funeral planning necessary for the circumstances immediately following a loved one's death. The FHD should understand who is in charge of the final decisions and who can facilitate discussions and agreements between family members, either by legal means or by family (next of kin, spouse, family by election, or children). Funeral arrangements require a plethora of decisions to be made during an emotional time and within an immediate time frame. The family's comfort and understanding regarding the decisions of who will be taking control of the body and what will happen to the remains is important (Lensing, 2001).

The Value of Funeral Preplanning

Preplanning a funeral is defined as the time when the patient, spouse or partner, children, caregivers, and legal and healthcare professionals meet to discuss the patient's wishes to be enacted at the time of his or her death (National Funeral Directors Association [NFDA], 2006). Discussions include costs, payment, traditional or nontraditional funeral rituals, prewritten obituaries, and acknowledgment of properties and disbursements. An existing advance care plan can later be used to influence medical events prior to death.

The following information is also important to gather and organize during the preplanning process.

A. Vital statistics and death certificate information
   1. Statistical and demographic information is required for the death certificate and includes the decedent's legal name, social security number (if not available, special arrangements are necessary), birth location, age at time of death, maiden name of parent, schools attended, time and place of death, cause of death, and legal next of kin.
   2. Four causes of death can be listed on death certificates: natural causes, homicide, suicide, and accident. Each category requires a different level of scrutiny by authorities such as the police, medical examiner, and local municipalities (NFDA, 2006).

B. Financial information
   1. The location and types of life insurance, savings accounts, stocks, bonds, investments, trusts, and debts owed should be ascertained.
   2. Insurance policies are reviewed to identify the beneficiary; in the case of a minor beneficiary, funds are not readily available for funeral expenses.

C. Disposition plans for the body
1. Understanding the plans for the body after death and who will become the "parties of association" (i.e., next of kin of the deceased or responsible parties) is important.
2. The following details and questions should be discussed with the patient and family.
    a) Is an autopsy to be requested?
    b) Is the body to be donated for science?
    c) Is full-body burial desired? If so, is embalming required, and will the body be placed above or below ground?
    d) Is cremation desired with or without full-body visitation prior to the funeral?
    e) If the body must be transported across state lines, the means of transportation and costs are discussed.
    f) If death should occur out of the country, the means and protocol to transport the body back into the designated state for burial is discussed (Weitzen, Teno, Fennell, & Mor, 2003).

D. Obituary information
1. The obituary is the A–Z of a person's life.
2. Obituaries published in newspapers and periodicals can be free if designated as an item of community interest.
3. The best obituary is one that is written ahead of time and agreed upon by the patient and his or her family.

E. Prepaid arrangements
1. Those planning the funeral must determine if arrangements are funded or nonfunded. Many families erroneously believe that funerals that were preplanned were also prepaid (NFDA, 2006).
2. Grief can be compounded when the surviving family discovers that plans have been instituted for the funeral but have not been paid for, and the financial burden now becomes their responsibility.

Strategies to Facilitate Funeral Planning

A. The following definitions are helpful to patients and families.
1. *Preneed:* The best gift that can be given to the survivors is the actual time it takes to plan for the events that follow one's death. Such needs involve advance care planning, envisioning plans for final acts of remembrance, and making plans for their financial management (NFDA, 2006).
2. *Preplanning:* Plans are documented and express the wishes of the person before death.
3. *Prefunding* and *prepaying:* Plans are associated with costs, with each cost detailing the options chosen, and each option is paid for in advance through

a safe, secure, reputable instrument (e.g., third-party holding accounts such as insurance policies, prefunded accounts, trust funds) (NFDA, 2006).

B. Many costs associated with funeral planning might be anticipated, such as payment for the site of the burial, opening and closing of the gravesite, choice of casket for burial or urn for cremation, choice of cemetery plot, type of hearse, limousine(s), security escort vehicles (particularly recommended in urban areas), flowers, costs for a reception, and any permits that may be required (such as for cremation). Some of these costs include "peace of mind" items; for example, a lined or unlined burial container may be chosen for sections of the country where flooding is a possibility (NFDA, 2006).

C. Identifying the patient's and family's needs concerning legal documents and advance directives is of primary importance. Advance directives are state-specific and should be carefully explained to the patient and family. Accessing www.caringinfo.org or the Caring Connections Helpline at 800-658-8898 can help to clarify state and federal legislation regarding advance directives.

Clinicians' Role in Funeral Planning

Clinicians can assist with answering patient and family questions about disease progression and estimated life expectancy and routinely discuss end-of-life care wishes. When the patient and family learn of a life-limiting prognosis, the clinician should advocate for the patient regarding specific wishes related to death and burial. Advocating these wishes to the healthcare team is a key palliative care nursing role (Lobar, Youngblut, & Brooten, 2006).

Clinicians should evaluate funeral planning needs for spiritual and cross-cultural care (Smith-Stoner, 2006). Conversations with the family regarding issues or rituals such as postmortem bathing and dressing of the body, anointing, and private meditation or prayer practices are necessary for providing culturally appropriate care. Muslim, Hindu, Jewish, Kurdish, or Hispanic patient populations may have additional concerns that need to be addressed by the interdisciplinary team (Hedayat, 2006; Sarhill, LeGrand, Islambouli, Davis, & Walsh, 2001). Clinicians should partner with the social workers and spiritual care providers to coordinate funeral planning assistance and bereavement services and communicate availability of bereavement support groups that include preparing children and teens for attending funerals and wakes (Hedayat).

Patient and Family Outcomes

A. The clinician will facilitate the process of funeral planning with appropriate healthcare teams and a funeral home director. These professionals will help the patient and family to accomplish the following.
   1. Advance directives are completed and their location(s) are identified.
   2. Pertinent cultural care issues and rituals are discussed and identified.

3. Plans for the body following death are known (i.e., full-body burial versus cremation).
4. Decisions regarding property disposition following death are explored.
5. Vital statistics, demographic information, and information for an obituary are accessible.

B. Discussions between the patient and family regarding the funding of the funeral and the various costs involved are facilitated.

C. *Preneed, preplanning, prefunding,* and *prepaying* are defined for the patient and family.

References

Angus, D.C., Barnato, A.E., Linde-Zwirble, W.T., Weissfeld, L.A., Watson, R.S., Rickert, T., et al. (2004). Use of intensive care at the end-of-life in the United States: An epidemiologic study. *Critical Care Medicine, 32,* 638–643.

Hedayat, K. (2006). When the spirit leaves: Childhood death, grieving, and bereavement in Islam. *Journal of Palliative Medicine, 9,* 1282–1291.

Lensing, V. (2001). Grief support: The role of the funeral service. *Journal of Loss and Trauma, 6,* 45–63.

Lobar, S.L., Youngblut, J.M., & Brooten, D. (2006). Cross-cultural beliefs, ceremonies, and rituals surrounding death of a loved one. *Pediatric Nursing, 32,* 44–50.

National Funeral Directors Association. (2006). *U.S. death statistics: 1960–2080.* Retrieved April 6, 2007, from http://www.nfda.org

Sarhill, N., LeGrand, S., Islambouli, R., Davis, M.P., & Walsh, D. (2001). The terminally ill Muslim: Death and dying from the Muslim perspective. *American Journal of Hospice and Palliative Care, 18,* 251–255.

SmithBucklin Corp., Market Research & Statistics Group. (2006, August). *2006 Cremation Association of North America (CANA) cremation container, disposition and service survey final results.* Retrieved April 6, 2007, from http://www.cremationassociation.org

Smith-Stoner, M. (2006). Phowa: End-of-life ritual prayers for Tibetan Buddhists. *Journal of Hospice and Palliative Nursing, 8,* 357–363.

Weitzen, S., Teno, J.M., Fennell, M., & Mor, V. (2003). Factors associated with site of death: A national study of where people die. *Medical Care, 41,* 323–335.

G

Grief and Bereavement

Grief and Bereavement

Marilyn O'Mallon, RN, MSN

Definitions

Grief

Grief is a universal human experience and is viewed as a normal response to loss and death. When considering the concept of grief in the palliative care setting, loss is associated with health and life (Hallenbeck, 2005). Additional losses might include the loss of body parts or function, functional status or changes in activities of daily living, career changes, relationships and changes in role identity, and finances associated with disability, all of which may intensify the grief experience for the patient and family. Grief involves personal internal processing and tasks that occur at the emotional, cognitive, and behavioral levels (Hallenbeck).

Anticipatory Grief

Anticipatory grief is the experience the patient and family undergo beginning with the initial diagnosis of a life-limiting illness and throughout the disease trajectory, death, and ultimately bereavement (Periyakoil, 2005). Anticipatory grief involves the process of reviewing one's life in preparation for the final separation from the world as perceived by each individual patient (Periyakoil). Patients often withdraw from family and friends during this important process. The clinician should identify withdrawal as a normal and important component of grief. Periods of sadness, crying, anxiety, and insomnia may occur during this period.

Complicated Grief

Complications that can occur from the normal grieving process include what is termed *complicated grief*. This form of grief can result whenever grief is unresolved, or it may represent a delay in the process of mourning or a grief response that persists over a prolonged period of time (i.e., greater than two years) (Dyer, 2006). Often, the grieving person stops functioning normally and may appear to be "stuck" in the process of finalizing or coming to the acceptance of a meaningful

The author would like to acknowledge Jerre Cory, MA, CSW, and Kim K. Kuebler, MN, RN, APRN-BC, for their contributions that remain unchanged from the first edition of this textbook.

loss. Complicated grief refers to the grief reactions or mourning processes that are not just unusual but abnormal in the sense of being unhealthy. Complicated grief is a state of being overwhelmed by emotions brought on by grief and accepting the loss. People experiencing severe complicated grief often need therapy to help to resolve the grieving process (Dyer).

Risk factors associated with complicated grief include sudden death; loss of a child; suicide, homicide, or accident; multiple losses; unresolved grief from a previous loss; and/or a poor support system (Egan & Arnold, 2003; McHale, 2005).

Bereavement

Bereavement is the acute phase of grief that is experienced by loved ones immediately following the actual death event. The American Institute for Preventive Medicine (1995) suggests that the normal period of grieving extends from one to three years. The length of bereavement is individualized and may last longer based upon individual circumstances. People from various cultural backgrounds may differ in their approach to grief and bereavement. (See Cultural Competence.) To facilitate healthy grieving, clinicians should consider individual religious and cultural beliefs of each patient and his or her family. Other factors that shape a patient or family response to loss include age, circumstances surrounding the death event, social network, history of other losses or traumatic events, and coping skills (McHale, 2005).

Family

Family is defined by the relationships that exist between individual family members (Kossmann & Bullrich, 1997). *Family* is defined by the U.S. Census Bureau as two or more individuals related by birth, adoption, marriage, or choice (Allen, Fine, & Demo, 2000). This definition "implies that families are defined primarily by long-term committed relationships, responsibilities, and ongoing support" (Demo, Aquilino, & Fine, 2005, p. 120). Each family member will have his or her own perception of loss and death that will affect the personal grief and bereavement experience. Advanced illness, dying, and death affect the family unit, an important consideration for the clinician who is providing care to the patient and family.

Specific Issues in Palliative Care

Coping with advanced illness and the associated symptomatology often intensify during the dying phase, and the actual death event can be one of the most difficult experiences in life for the patient and family. Family members may encounter somatic experiences as a result of the emotional burden associated with grief and bereavement, including fatigue, muscle weakness, loss of appetite, insomnia, pain, and nervousness (Lindemann, 1994; Vena, Kuebler, & Schrader, 2005).

Psychoemotional experiences often include waves of vague sensations of illness or physical discomfort accompanied by feelings of loneliness, emptiness, abandonment, fear, anxiety, and a sense of being lost or uncertain about the future

(Vena et al., 2005). Significant lymphocyte suppression has been reported in the bereaved one month after the death event. This physical reaction in the bereaved seems to correlate with the death event itself (Schleifer, Keller, Camerino, Thornton, & Stein, 1983; Vena et al.). Suppressed immunity following the death of a spouse or loved one may be related to increased morbidity and mortality in the bereaved (Schleifer et al.; Vena et al.).

Strategies to Promote Interventions in Palliative Care

A. Grief and bereavement interventions that clinicians can utilize when caring for patients and their loved ones during the dying process can help to support a healthy normal dying event and reduce a difficult or complicated grief and bereavement experience (McHale, 2005). Interventions include providing the patient and family with specific palliative and end-of-life care services that involve an interdisciplinary team who can help to support the complex needs that accompany death and dying (e.g., medical, nursing, psychosocial, spiritual, financial).

B. The bedside clinician should evaluate for and assess potential risk factors that may precipitate a complicated grieving process leading to a prolonged and unhealthy bereavement phase. Assisting the patient and family with meaningful events that can bring closure is important. The following interventions can assist in healthy life closure.

1. Assess and evaluate important and meaningful events that the patient would like to accomplish prior to death.
2. Help to provide a realistic framework for the patient and family related to the physical demands associated with accomplishing tasks that may not be attainable.
3. Encourage open and direct communication between the patient and family.
4. Provide education on symptom management to the patient and family to ensure optimal symptom relief and quality of life.
5. Provide referrals to specific disciplines to support the physical, emotional, and spiritual needs of the patient and family.

Evaluating the Evidence

A. **Level III—low level of evidence**

The literature does not represent data from randomized controlled trials that evaluate the effect of grief and bereavement on human health. However, sufficient evidence exists regarding the vagueness and ambiguity of the terms and definitions used to describe grief and bereavement. The literature provides evidence on individual and unique responses associated with grief and bereavement, but evidence is limited to identify specific practice interventions leading to positive patient and family outcomes (Cope, 2003).

B. Approximately one-third of bereaved people develop problems that require professional assistance, including an increased use of tobacco, alcohol, sedatives, and antianxiety medications (Pietcuszka, 1992). The use of nonprescriptive drugs and alcohol as a coping strategy to combat the impact of grief is not a healthy strategy and requires prompt attention and referral to appropriate professionals (Asaro & Clements, 2005). Clinicians should monitor for ineffective coping strategies during the bereavement process (Kissane, McKenzie, & Bloch, 1997).

Patient and Family Outcomes

A. The patient obtains final and effective life closure with self and meaningful relationships.

B. Open and effective communication patterns between the patient and family are maintained.

C. Patient and family receive adequate information about available resources and interventions throughout the dying process.

D. Patient and family exhibit healthy, normal reactions to loss and death throughout the grief and bereavement process.

References

Allen, K.R., Fine, M.A., & Demo, D.H. (2000). An overview of family diversity: Controversies, questions, and values. In D.H. Demo, K.R. Allen, & M.A. Fine (Eds.), *Handbook of family diversity* (pp. 1–14). New York: Oxford University Press.

American Institute for Preventive Medicine. (1995). *Grief/bereavement.* Retrieved May 20, 2007, from http://www.healthy.net/scr/Article.asp?Id=1829

Asaro, M.R., & Clements, P.T. (2005). Homicide bereavement: A family affair. *Journal of Forensic Nursing, 1,* 101–105, 128.

Cope, D. (2003). Evidence-based practice: Making it happen in your clinical setting. *Clinical Journal of Oncology Nursing, 7,* 97–98.

Demo, D.H., Aquilino, W.S., & Fine, M.A. (2005). Family composistion and family transitions. In V.L. Bengtson, A.C. Acock, K.R. Allen, P. Dilworth-Anderson, & D.M. Klein (Eds.), *Sourcebook of family theory and research* (pp. 119–142). Thousand Oaks, CA: Sage Publications.

Dyer, K.A. (2006). *Definition of complicated grief, mourning or bereavement.* Retrieved February 15, 2008, from http://www.dying.about.com/od/glossary/g/comp_grief.htm

Egan, K.A., & Arnold, R.L. (2003). Grief and bereavement care. *American Journal of Nursing, 103*(9), 42–53.

Hallenbeck, J. (2005). *Fast facts and concepts #32: Grief and bereavement* (2nd ed.). Retrieved May 20, 2007, from http://www.eperc.mcw.edu/fastFact/ff_32.htm

Kissane, D.W., McKenzie, D.P., & Bloch, S. (1997). Family coping and bereavement outcome. *Palliative Medicine, 11,* 191–201.

Kossmann, M.R., & Bullrich, S. (1997). Systematic chaos: Self-organizing systems and the process of change. In F. Masterpasqua & P.A. Perna (Eds.), *The psychological meaning of chaos: Translating theory into practice* (pp. 199–223). Washington, DC: American Psychological Association.

Lindemann, E. (1994). Symptomology and management of acute grief: 1944. *American Journal of Psychiatry, 151*(Suppl. 6), 155–160.

McHale, H. (2005). Grief and bereavement. In K. Kuebler, M. Davis, & C. Moore (Eds.), *Palliative practices: An interdisciplinary approach* (pp. 379–400). St. Louis, MO: Elsevier Saunders.

Periyakoil, V.J. (2005). *Fast facts and concepts #043: Is it grief or depression?* (2nd ed.). Retrieved May 20, 2007, from http://www.eperc.mcw.edu/FastFactPDF/Concept%20043.pdf

Pietcuszka, F.M. (1992). Management of bereavement in the elderly. *Physician Assistant, 16,* 37–44.

Schleifer, S.J., Keller, S.E., Camerino, M., Thornton, J.C., & Stein, M. (1983). Suppression of lymphocyte stimulation following bereavement. *JAMA, 250,* 374–377.

Vena, C., Kuebler, K., & Schrader, S. (2005). The dying process. In K. Kuebler, M. Davis, & C. Moore (Eds.), *Palliative practices: An interdisciplinary approach* (pp. 335–368). St. Louis, MO: Elsevier Saunders.

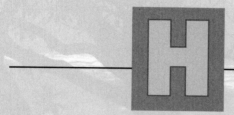

Hiccups

Hiccups

Jerald M. Andry, PharmD, MSc

Definitions

Hiccup, also called *singultus,* is a characteristic sound that is produced by the involuntary contraction of the diaphragm and intercostal muscles followed by rapid closure of the glottis. Hiccups lasting up to 48 hours are referred to as a hiccup bout and are considered acute. Hiccups lasting longer than 48 hours are referred to as persistent hiccups, and those lasting for more than two months are considered intractable (Souadjian & Cain, 1968).

Pathophysiology and Etiology

Hiccups are mediated by the phrenic and vagus nerves and a central reflex center. The central mediator is thought to involve the respiratory centers, the phrenic nerve nuclei, the reticular part of the brain stem, and the hypothalamus. More than a hundred causes for hiccups are likely to exist, with the most common being gastrointestinal in nature. Additionally, men are more likely to experience hiccups than women (Cymet, 2002). The common causes of hiccups can be classified into one of the following categories.
- Conditions that cause vagus and phrenic nerve irritation or diaphragm irritation (e.g., gastric distention, gastritis, ulcers, gastroesophageal reflux disease, bowel obstruction)
- Central nervous system disorders (e.g., trauma, multiple sclerosis, encephalitis)
- Metabolic disorders (e.g., uremia, hypokalemia, hypocalcemia, alcohol ingestion or abuse, diabetes mellitus)
- Psychogenic factors (e.g., stress, anxiety)
- Drugs (e.g., parenteral corticosteroids, barbiturates, benzodiazepines, chemotherapeutic agents, pain medications)
- Infectious disorders (e.g., influenza, herpes zoster, malaria, tuberculosis)

The author would like to acknowledge Kimberly A. Zielke, MD, for her contributions that remain unchanged from the first edition of this textbook.

- Idiopathic causes

(Esper, 2007; Smith & Busracamwongs, 2003; Twycross & Regnarol, 1998)

In the palliative care patient, gastric distention is likely the most common cause of hiccups, accounting for up to 95% of cases (Twycross & Regnarol, 1998).

Manifestations

Persistent hiccups:
- Fatigue
- Sleep disturbances
- Respiratory alkalosis in tracheotomized patients
- Nausea
- Abdominal discomfort

Management

A. Treatment of hiccups should be directed at the underlying cause if one can be identified. If medications are identified as the possible cause, discontinuation of medication should be considered. However, the cause of hiccups often cannot be identified or addressed clinically; thus, general treatments should be considered.

B. Pharmacologic interventions
   1. Medications used to treat hiccups include drugs and muscle relaxants that target phrenic/vagal stimulation, reduction in gastric distention, and central suppression of the hiccup reflex through interactions with gamma-aminobutyric acid and dopamine transmission. Currently, the only U.S. Food and Drug Administration-approved medication to treat intractable hiccups is chlorpromazine. Other medications that have been used to treat hiccups are listed as follows.
   2. **Level II—moderate level of evidence**
      (Esper, 2007; Hernandez et al., 2004; Marechal, Berghmans, & Sculier, 2003; Moro, Sironi, Berardi, Beretta, & Labianca, 2005; Smith & Busracamwongs, 2003)
      a) Simethicone-containing antacids (Maalox-Plus®) ($)—5–10 ml four times daily before or after meals and at bedtime, or 25 mg/5 ml suspension as needed
      b) Chlorpromazine (Thorazine®) ($)—25–50 mg three or four times daily. If symptoms persist for two to three days, give 25–50 mg (1–2 ml) via intramuscular injection. Should symptoms persist, use slow IV infusion with patient flat in bed: 25–50 mg (1–2 ml) in 500–1,000 ml of saline. Follow blood pressure and sedation closely.
      c) Baclofen (Lioresal®) ($)—5–20 mg po two or three times daily
      d) Carbamazepine (Tegretol®) ($$)—200 mg po three or four times daily

e) Gabapentin (Neurontin®) ($$)—300–400 mg po three times daily

f) Haloperidol (Haldol®) ($)—5 mg IV every six hours initially and/or 1–4 mg subcutaneous (SC) three times daily

g) Methylphenidate (Ritalin®) ($$)—5 mg po twice daily

h) Metoclopramide (Reglan®) ($$)—10 mg IV over two minutes, followed by 10 mg po three to four times daily

i) Midazolam ($$)—IV or SC 30–120 mg per 24 hours. Used in patients who are close to death and have persistent distressing hiccups.

C. Nonpharmacologic interventions

  1. Nonpharmacologic interventions have usually been attempted by patients prior to contacting a healthcare professional.

  2. **Level III—low level of evidence**

    (Cymet, 2002; Dobelle, 1999; Esper, 2007; Smith & Busracamwongs, 2003)

    a) Holding one's breath

    b) Compression of the nose while swallowing

    c) Breathing into a paper bag

    d) Hypnosis

    e) Valsalva maneuver (forcibly exhaling against closed lips and pinched nose, thus forcing air into the middle ear if the Eustachian tube is open)

    f) Breathing pacemakers

    g) Acupuncture

    h) Biting a lemon

    i) Eating a teaspoon of sugar

    j) Drinking peppermint water

    k) Vagus nerve stimulation

    l) Diaphragmatic pacing electrodes

  3. Little evidence exists to suggest that one intervention is better than another, as many of the techniques reported are anecdotal. Surgical methods (phrenic nerve ablation) are recommended only in severe intractable cases.

Patient Outcomes

A. Hiccups are resolved.

B. Patient's comfort is restored.

C. Patient experiences less distress.

References

Cymet, T.C. (2002). Retrospective analysis of hiccups in patients at a community hospital from 1995–2000. *Journal of the National Medical Association, 94*, 480–483.

Dobelle, W.H. (1999). Use of breathing pacemakers to suppress intractable hiccups of up to thirteen years duration. *American Society for Artificial Internal Organs Journal, 45*, 524–525.

Esper, P. (2007). Hiccups. In K.K. Kuebler, D.E. Heidrich, & P. Esper (Eds.), *Palliative and end-of-life care: Clinical practice guidelines* (2nd ed., pp. 411–416). St. Louis, MO: Elsevier Saunders.

Hernandez, J.L., Pajaron, M., Garcia-Regata, O., Jimenez, V., Gonzalez-Macias, J., & Ramos-Estebanez, C. (2004). Gabapentin for intractable hiccup. *American Journal of Medicine, 117,* 279–281.

Marechal, R., Berghmans, T., & Sculier, P. (2003). Successful treatment of intractable hiccup with methylphenidate in a lung cancer patient. *Supportive Care in Cancer, 11,* 126–128.

Moro, C., Sironi, P., Berardi, E., Beretta, G., & Labianca, R. (2005). Midazolam for long-term treatment of intractable hiccup. *Journal of Pain and Symptom Management, 29,* 221–223.

Smith, H.S., & Busracamwongs, A. (2003). Management of hiccups in the palliative care population. *American Journal of Hospice and Palliative Care, 20,* 149–154.

Souadjian, J.V., & Cain, J.C. (1968). Intractable hiccup: Etiologic factors in 220 cases. *Postgraduate Medicine, 43*(2), 72–77.

Twycross, R., & Regnarol, C. (1998). Dysphagia, dyspepsia, and hiccups. In D. Doyle, G.W.C. Hanks, & N. MacDonald (Eds.), *Oxford textbook of palliative medicine* (2nd ed., pp. 508–510). New York: Oxford University Press.

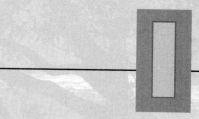

Infection

Insomnia

Infection

Linda A. Upchurch, MSN, ANP-BC, CHPN, Jill R. Nelson, RN, MSN, APRN-BC, and James C. Pace, DSN, RN, MDiv, ANP-BC, FAANP

Definition

Infection is the invasion of the body by foreign organisms that disrupt host homeostasis. Some bacterial infections, similar to those that contribute to pneumonia, respond well to antimicrobial interventions. Antimicrobials are antibiotics or antifungal agents. Viral infections, such as those that cause the common cold, are self-limited and will not respond to antimicrobials. For palliative care purposes, antimicrobials typically are used to control symptoms related to active or suspected infections (Reinbolt, Shenk, White, & Navari, 2005).

Pathophysiology and Etiology

Patients with advanced illness are at a heightened risk for infection. This increased risk is a result of a number of factors, including but not limited to "impaired immunity of multiple possible etiologies, malnutrition, asthenia, decreased level of consciousness, immobility, failure of host barriers, and the use of foreign bodies" (Nagy-Agren & Haley, 2002, pp. 64–65). One-third of terminally ill patients experience an infection in the last stages of disease (Vitetta, Kenner, & Sali, 2000). Frequent infections that accompany advanced illness include urinary tract, respiratory, and skin/subcutaneous infections (White, Kuhlenschmidt, Vancura, & Navari, 2003).

Manifestations

Manifestations are dependent on the site of infection and may include the following.
- Fever
- Cough
- Disorientation
- Dyspnea

The authors would like to acknowledge Peg Esper, MSN, MSA, RN, AOCN®, APRN-BC, for her contribution that remains unchanged from the first edition of this textbook.

- Dysuria
- Urinary frequency
- Hypotension
- Odynophagia
- Pain
- Skin rash or discoloration
- Sputum production

(Reinbolt et al., 2005)

Management

A. The priority of management is to prevent infection when possible. Measures to prevent infection include the following.
  1. Avoid contact with known pathogens or carriers.
  2. Perform meticulous skin and wound care.
  3. Optimize functional physical activity.
  4. Regularly change indwelling catheters.
  5. Implement antibiotic prophylaxis, when appropriate.
  6. Encourage the patient to practice regular oral hygiene.
  7. Encourage adequate nutrition, when possible.

B. The use of antimicrobials in the palliative care setting is complex. Several factors require consideration before initiation of treatment, including disease status, body function, pain and other symptoms, and to include patient/family goals of treatment (Nagy-Agren & Haley, 2002). Infection control is appropriate for comfort and palliative symptom management; however, the use of antibiotics may not affect overall patient survival (Reinbolt et al., 2005; White et al., 2003).

C. Death is not imminent.
  1. **Level I—high level of evidence**
     a) Antipyretic administration ($)—acetaminophen, aspirin, or ibuprofen (Rhiner & Slatkin, 2005)
     b) Analgesics for general discomfort and headache ($)—acetaminophen, aspirin, or ibuprofen (Paice & Fine, 2006)
     c) Treatments for suspected respiratory tract infection—Usual causes may include *Streptococcus pneumoniae, Haemophilus influenzae, Moraxella catarrhalis,* and group A *Streptococcus* (Institute for Clinical Systems Improvement, 2007).
        (1) Broad-spectrum antibiotics ($–$$$)—amoxicillin (Amoxil®), azithromycin (Zithromax®), and trimethoprim/sulfamethoxazole (Bactrim®) (Institute for Clinical Systems Improvement, 2007)
        (2) Consider the use of an antibiotic in liquid form for patients with dysphagia.
        (3) Suspected *Pneumocystis jiroveci* pneumonia (formerly *Pneumocystis carinii* pneumonia should be treated with trimethoprim/

sulfamethoxazole DS. Administer two tablets po every eight hours for 21 days. An alternative treatment is dapsone administered at a dosage of 100 mg po every 24 hours with trimethoprim 5 mg/kg po three times a day for 21 days (Gilbert, Moellering, Eliopoulos, & Sande, 2006).

 d) Treatment for urinary tract infection (UTI)—Usual causes may include *Escherichia coli, Staphylococcus saprophyticus,* and enterococci (Edmunds & Mayhew, 2004).

 (1) Encourage increased fluid intake. In the past, patients have been encouraged to drink cranberry juice to increase urine acidity. However, current research suggests the benefits are related to prevention of bacterial adherence to the bladder (Martino et al., 2006).

 (2) Antibiotics ($–$$)—UTIs often can be treated with a short course of antibiotics, but recurrence is common, and maintenance dosing may be required. Typical antibiotic treatments for UTI include ciprofloxacin (Cipro®), trimethoprim/sulfamethoxazole (Bactrim), cephalexin (Keflex®), ampicillin, and nitrofurantoin (Macrodantin®) (maintenance) (Edmunds & Mayhew, 2004).

 (3) Change indwelling urinary catheters on a regular basis using aseptic techniques.

 (4) Encourage regular cleansing around the catheter insertion site.

 (5) Review procedure for intermittent self-catheterization.

 (6) To ease pain, itching, burning, urgency, and frequency, administer phenazopyridine (Pyridium®) ($)—100–200 mg po three times daily, after meals usually for two to three days. Alert the patient and family that urine and tears may have an orange discoloration (Edmunds & Mayhew, 2004).

 2. **Level II—moderate level of evidence**
   a) Fungal or yeast infections
   (1) Keep site clean and dry if outside of oral cavity.
   (2) Topical or oral antifungal agents ($–$$)
   (a) For oral candidiasis, nystatin suspension (100,000 U/ml) 15 ml swish and swallow six times daily, or clotrimazole troche 10 mg held in the mouth 15–30 minutes three times daily
   (b) For esophageal candidiasis, fluconazole (Diflucan®) 200 mg po the first day, then 100 mg po once daily for two to three weeks (Boswell, 2006)
   (3) Monitor for recurrence.
   b) Wound infections (See Skin Lesions.)

D. Death is imminent.
   Level I—high level of evidence
   1. The burden of treatment may outweigh the benefit if life expectancy is limited (Van der Steen, Ooms, Ader, Ribbe, & Van der Wal, 2002). Anti-

biotics may be appropriate when infection interferes with patient comfort (Nagy-Agren & Haley, 2002).

2. When death is imminent, comfort is the priority, and the following measures should be instituted.
   a) Manage fever and chills (Rhiner & Slatkin, 2005).
   b) Manage dyspnea and cough (use of oxygen, opiates, or anxiolytics). (See Cough and Dyspnea.)
   c) Manage drainage or odor from infection, wounds, or catheter sites. (See Skin Lesions.)
   d) Provide analgesic support as needed. (See Pain.)

Patient Outcomes

A. Patient and caregivers understand the signs and symptoms of infection and report symptoms to the clinician.

B. The infection is treated per the plan of care, which includes providing assessment, intervention, and evaluation.

C. When death is imminent, comfort is maintained.

References

Boswell, S.L. (2006). Approach to the patient with HIV infection. In A.H. Goroll & A.G. Mulley (Eds.), *Primary care medicine: Office evaluation and management of the adult patient* (5th ed., pp. 88–89). Philadelphia: Lippincott Williams & Wilkins.

Edmunds, M.W., & Mayhew, M.S. (2004). *Pharmacology for the primary care provider* (2nd ed.). St. Louis, MO: Mosby.

Gilbert, D.N., Moellering, R.C., Jr., Eliopoulos, G.M., & Sande, M.A. (2006). *The Sanford guide to antimicrobial therapy* (36th ed.). Sperryville, VA: Antimicrobial Therapy.

Institute for Clinical Systems Improvement. (2007, January). *Diagnosis and treatment of respiratory illness in children and adults*. Retrieved June 12, 2007, from http://www.guideline.gov/summary/ summary.aspx?ss=15&doc_id=10622&nbr=5564

Martino, P., Agniel, R., David, K., Templer, C., Gaillard, J.L., Denys, P., et al. (2006). Reduction of *Escherichia coli* adherence to uroepithelial bladder cells after consumption of cranberry juice: A double-blind randomized placebo-controlled cross-over trial. *World Journal of Urology, 24,* 21–27.

Nagy-Agren, S., & Haley, H.B. (2002). Management of infections in palliative care patients with advanced cancer. *Journal of Pain and Symptom Management, 24,* 64–70.

Paice, J.A., & Fine, P.G. (2006). Pain at the end of life. In B.R. Ferrell & N. Coyle (Eds.), *Textbook of palliative nursing* (pp. 133–134). New York: Oxford University Press.

Reinbolt, R.E., Shenk, A.M., White, P.H., & Navari, R.M. (2005). Symptomatic treatment of infections in patients with advanced cancer receiving hospice care. *Journal of Pain and Symptom Management, 30,* 175–182.

Rhiner, M., & Slatkin, N. (2006). Pruritus, fever and sweats. In B.R. Ferrell & N. Coyle (Eds.), *Textbook of palliative nursing* (pp. 345–363). New York: Oxford University Press.

Van der Steen, J.T., Ooms, M.E., Ader, H.J., Ribbe, M.W., & Van der Wal, G. (2002). Withholding antibiotic treatment in pneumonia patients with dementia: A quantitative observational study. *Archives of Internal Medicine, 162,* 1753–1760.

Vitetta, L., Kenner, D., & Sali, A. (2000). Bacterial infections in terminally ill hospice patients. *Journal of Pain and Symptom Management, 20,* 326–334.

White, P.H., Kuhlenschmidt, H.L., Vancura, B.G., & Navari, R.M. (2003). Antimicrobial use in patients with advanced cancer receiving hospice care. *Journal of Pain and Symptom Management, 25,* 438–443.

Insomnia

Kim Anne Pickett, MS, CRNP

Definition

Insomnia is described as the subjective complaint of inadequate sleep, including difficulty initiating or maintaining sleep, frequent awakening, or poor quality of sleep. The amount of sleep each person requires varies greatly but can range from as little as 4 hours to as many as 11 hours daily, with an average at about 7 hours per day (Simon & Sunseri, 2003; Wolkove, Elkholy, Baltzan, & Palayew, 2007). Insomnia occurs frequently in the palliative care setting and is often an underreported symptom.

Pathophysiology and Etiology

Insomnia may be classified as primary (i.e., no identifiable cause) or secondary, which can be attributed to an underlying cause. The physiologic process involved is dependent on the etiology of insomnia and may be multifactorial. Uncontrolled symptoms, such as pain, dyspnea, nausea, constipation, diarrhea, pruritus, and cough, contribute to the inability to sleep. Certain medications, such as phenytoin, diuretics, caffeine, bronchodilators (i.e., beta agonists), corticosteroids, and selective serotonin reuptake inhibitors (SSRIs); treatments such as chemotherapy and radiation; and lifestyle habits that include smoking and alcohol use are all risk factors for precipitating insomnia. Psychosocial issues, such as anxiety, fear, agitation, depression, and confusion, may contribute to the inability to sleep (Graci, 2005; Simon & Sunseri, 2003; Vena, 2007; Wolkove et al., 2007). Insomnia occurs frequently in older adults and in patients with advanced illness and can have a negative effect on the patient's quality of life and functional status (Kvale & Shuster, 2006).

Manifestations

- Difficulty getting to sleep
- Frequent waking during the night

The author would like to acknowledge Peg Esper, MSN, MSA, RN, AOCN®, APRN-BC, for her contribution that remains unchanged from the first edition of this textbook.

- Early morning awakening
- Fatigue
- Decreased daytime functioning and cognition
- Mental status changes, such as confusion, delirium, or agitation
- Anxiety related to intrusive thoughts, fear of the unknown, or distressing dreams (Vena, 2007)

Management

A. Management of insomnia should focus on examining the cause and contributing factors precipitating the patient's inability to sleep. Managing the underlying pathology, such as pain, dyspnea, headaches, frequent urination, nausea, or anxiety, is important. Feelings of sadness and isolation are not easily relieved with benzodiazepines; therefore, important and personal psychosocial issues or concerns must be addressed (Wright, 2002). In addition to a thorough medical history, a current and past sleep history should be assessed to evaluate the patient's sleep patterns. Sleep history, hours per night engaged in sleep, sleep quality, and whether the condition is an acute or chronic occurrence, as well as previous treatments and outcomes, are all important to review. The use of a sleep diary or a structured questionnaire can be an effective way to obtain data and to identify patterns (Kvale & Shuster, 2006; Simon & Sunseri, 2003; Taylor, Vazquez, & Campbell, 2006).

B. Death is not imminent.
  1. **Level II—moderate level of evidence**
     a) Nonpharmacologic interventions
         (1) Cognitive behavioral therapy (CBT)—CBT combines cognitive therapy with strategies to improve sleep habits. Although CBT may be difficult to use in certain palliative care populations and usually is administered by a psychotherapist, strong evidence exists for its efficacy, especially with long-term use. Basic principles of CBT include but are not limited to psychotherapy augmented by one or more of the following techniques (Edinger, Wohlgemuth, Radtke, Marsh, & Quillian, 2001; Kvale & Shuster, 2006; Vena, 2007).
             (a) Relaxation therapy—The use of guided imagery, relaxation tapes, and progressive muscle relaxation provides a comfortable environment conducive to sleep.
             (b) Sleep restriction, sleep hygiene, and stimulus control—The patient promotes sleep by limiting the amount of time spent in the bed, getting out of bed during extended awakenings, minimizing daytime napping, and establishing a standard wake- up time.
         (2) Chronotherapy and phototherapy treatment of circadian rhythm disturbances—These treatments have not been studied in the palliative care setting.

      (3) Studies regarding nonpharmacologic treatments are limited at this level.

   b) Pharmacologic interventions

      (1) If CBT alone is not effective, the use of medications may be beneficial. Although hypnotics and benzodiazepines have been studied extensively, no strong evidence exists for the use of hypnotics in the palliative care population (Hirst & Sloan, 2002).

      (2) The following medications may be beneficial short-term therapy (less than 14 days). The lowest effective dose should be used in older adults and palliative care patients because of the likelihood of drug-drug interactions and polypharmacy.

         (a) Benzodiazepines

            i) Temazepam (Restoril®) ($)—15–30 mg po at bedtime as needed

            ii) Triazolam (Halcion®) ($)—0.125–0.25 mg po at bedtime as needed

         (b) Hypnotics ($$–$$$)

            i) Zolpidem (Ambien®) ($$)—5–10 mg po at bedtime as needed

            ii) Zaleplon (Sonata®) ($$$)—5–10 mg po at bedtime as needed

            iii) Eszopiclone (Lunesta®) ($$$)—1–3 mg po at bedtime as needed

      (3) Antianxiety agents ($–$$) (See Anxiety.)

      (4) Antidepressants ($–$$) (See Depression.)

      (5) When prescribing agents, practitioners should determine if the problem is primarily related to sleep onset or sleep maintenance. Zolpidem or zaleplon should be considered for patients who experience sleep onset insomnia. Patients with sleep maintenance insomnia may benefit from either an intermediate-acting benzodiazepine, such as temazepam, or the hypnotic eszopiclone (Nichols, Alper, & Milkin, 2007; Taylor et al., 2006).

2. **Level III—low level of evidence**

   a) Nonprescription medications (Chokroverty, 2007; Taylor et al., 2006; Vena, 2007)

      (1) Supplements/herbal products (melatonin, valerian extract)—Limited evidence exists regarding the safety and efficacy of these over-the-counter medications. They may have multiple drug interactions, and screening for the use of these medications and prior outcomes is important when obtaining the sleep history.

      (2) Antihistamines (diphenhydramine, hydroxyzine)—No strong evidence exists for use for insomnia, but antihistamines may be helpful and readily available for the patient or caregiver to initiate for use on a short-term basis. They may have side effects of daytime sedation, dizziness, dry mouth, and constipation, which require close monitoring.

    b) Nonpharmacologic interventions (Vena, 2007)
       (1) Encourage meaningful interactions during daytime hours to minimize patient boredom and loneliness.
       (2) Establish a bedtime routine.
       (3) Avoid intake of stimulant foods or beverages for at least three hours before bedtime.
       (4) Provide optimum comfort in the room (use lighting and sounds that are preferred by the patient).
       (5) Provide relaxation and comfort in the form of prayer, meditation, aromatherapy, or massage.
       (6) Provide counseling to deal with underlying fears and/or anticipatory grieving.
       (7) Position the patient on his or her side or elevate the head of the bed slightly to enhance sleep.

C. Death is imminent.
  1. Focus on maintaining the patient's immediate comfort.
  2. During the last few days to weeks of life, the patient may begin to sleep with increasing frequency. The family's concerns should be acknowledged regarding this normal process.
  3. Terminal agitation, anxiety, fear, pain, urinary retention, and constipation should undergo routine evaluation and assessment.

Patient Outcomes

A. Satisfactory periods of sustained sleep are attained.

B. Rest is adequate to allow participation in meaningful activities.

References

Chokroverty, S. (2007). *Evaluation and treatment of insomnia*. Retrieved April 24, 2007, from http://www.uptodateonline.com

Edinger, J.D., Wohlgemuth, W.K., Radtke, R.A., Marsh, G.R., & Quillian, R.E. (2001). Cognitive behavioral therapy for treatment of chronic primary insomnia: A randomized controlled trial. *JAMA, 285,* 1856–1864.

Graci, G. (2005). Pathogenesis and management of cancer-related insomnia. *Journal of Supportive Oncology, 3,* 349–359.

Hirst, A., & Sloan, R. (2002). Benzodiazepines and related drugs for insomnia in palliative care. *Cochrane Database of Systematic Reviews 2002,* Issue 4. Art. No.: CD003346. DOI: 10.1002/14651858. CD 003346.

Kvale, E.A., & Shuster, J.L. (2006). Sleep disturbance in supportive care of cancer: A review. *Journal of Palliative Medicine, 9,* 437–450.

Nichols, J., Alper, C., & Milkin, T. (2007). Strategies for the management of insomnia: An update on pharmacologic therapies. *Formulary, 42,* 86–98.

Simon, R.P., & Sunseri, M.J. (2003). Disorders of sleep and arousal. In L. Goldman & D. Ausiello (Eds.), *Cecil textbook of medicine* (22nd ed., pp. 2277–2281). Philadelphia: Saunders.

Taylor, J.R., Vazquez, C.M., & Campbell, K.M. (2006). Pharmacologic management of chronic insomnia. *Southern Medical Journal, 99,* 1373–1377.

Vena, C. (2007). Sleep. In K.K. Kuebler, D.E. Heidrich, & P. Esper (Eds.), *Palliative and end-of-life care: Clinical practice guidelines* (2nd ed., pp. 111–129). St. Louis, MO: Elsevier Saunders.

Wolkove, N., Elkholy, O., Baltzan, M., & Palayew, M. (2007). Sleep and aging: 1. Sleep disorders commonly found in older people. *Canadian Medical Association Journal, 176,* 1299–1304.

Wright, J.B. (2002). Depression and other common symptoms. In B.M. Kinzbrunner, N.J. Weinreb, & J.S. Policzer (Eds.), *20 common problems in end-of-life care* (pp. 221–241). New York: McGraw-Hill.

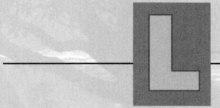

Lymphedema

Lymphedema

Sheila H. Ridner, PhD, RN, ACNP

Definition

Lymphedema is a condition in which excessive fluid and protein accumulate in the extravascular and interstitial spaces (Rockson, 2001). Lymphedema can either be primary, caused by genetic and familial lymphatic abnormalities, or secondary, caused by trauma to the lymph system from cancer treatment, surgery, or accidental injury (Petrek, Pressman, & Smith, 2000; Williams, Franks, & Moffatt, 2005).

Pathophysiology and Etiology

Lymphedema occurs when the lymphatic system cannot accept or transport lymph into the circulatory system (Browse, Burnand, & Mortimer, 2003). Patients in the palliative care setting can experience worsening of preexisting lymphedema or develop new-onset lymphedema. A number of factors contribute to the worsening or development of lymphedema (Browse et al., 2003; Guyton & Hall, 2006; Ridner, 2002).

- Tumor bulk can block lymph nodes or drainage pathways.
- Infection may cause lymph structures and surrounding tissue to fibrose and diminish lymphatic transport capacity.
- Immobility in patients who are actively dying reduces the movement of fluid through lymphatic channels.
- Surgical removal of nodes and tissue and tied-off lymph vessels can obstruct drainage channels and diminish carrying capacity.
- Scarring and fibrosis of lymph structures and surrounding tissues secondary to radiation treatment can obstruct lymphatic drainage, damage the lumens of lymphatic trunks, and alter the cell membrane of lymphatic vessels.

The author would like to acknowledge Peg Esper, MSN, MSA, RN, AOCN®, APRN-BC, for her contribution that remains unchanged from the first edition of this textbook.

Manifestations

Clinical Presentation
- Swelling of affected limb or area
- Heaviness
- Burning
- Pain
- Warmth
- Erythema
- Skin cracked or oozing clear fluid
- Tightness
- Fatigue
- Decreased mobility

(Armer & Ridner, 2007)

Differential Diagnoses
- Myxedema
- Lipedema
- Deep vein thrombosis
- Chronic venous insufficiency
- Cancer recurrence or spread
- Cellulitis
- Other infections

Management

A. Conduct a thorough history and physical examination (Armer & Ridner, 2007).
   1. History
      a) The course of lymphedema, including onset (new or preexisting) and location(s)
      b) Medications and medical treatment (e.g., radiation, surgery, antibiotic therapy)
      c) Symptoms
      d) Current lymphedema management strategies
      e) Ability of patient or caregiver to provide at-home care for lymphedema
   2. Physical
      a) Location and degree of swelling (measure volume if possible)
      b) Skin assessment
      c) Signs of infection

B. Death is not imminent.
   1. **Level I—high level of evidence**
      a) Measurement of volume ($–$$$$)
         (1) Water displacement ($) (Megens, Harris, Kim-Sing, & McKenzie, 2001)
         (2) Circumferential measurement of limb volume ($) (Armer, 2005)
         (3) Infrared perometry ($$$$) (Ridner, Montgomery, Hepworth, Stewart, & Armer, 2007)
         (4) Bioelectrical impedance ($$$$) (Ridner et al., 2007)
      b) Volume reduction ($–$$$$)
         (1) No approved or recommended pharmacologic approach to volume reduction exists.
         (2) Do not use diuretics, as they will not be beneficial for lymphedema.

      (3) If heart failure or venous incompetence is also present, then diuretics may improve overall patient comfort (Twycross, 2000).

   c) Nonpharmacologic interventions

      (1) Complex decongestive physiotherapy ($$) (if the patient can tolerate this intense approach to the management of lymphedema) (Hamner & Fleming, 2007; Hinrichs et al., 2004)

        (a) Skin care

        (b) Massage

        (c) Bandaging

        (d) Exercise

      (2) Manual lymph drainage ($$)—The patient and caregivers can be instructed by a physical therapist or a lymphedema specialist to perform this procedure (Finlay, 1999; McNeely et al., 2004).

      (3) Compression garments ($–$$)—bandages or compression stockings (Badger, Peacock, & Mortimer, 2000)

      (4) Compression devices ($$$$) (Wilburn, Wilburn, & Rockson, 2006)

   d) Treatment for lymphedema-related infection ($)

      (1) Streptococcal—penicillin V 0.5 g every six hours

      (2) Staphylococcal, etiology uncertain—dicloxacillin 0.5 g every six hours

      (3) For patients who are sensitive to penicillin—erythromycin 0.5 g every six hours (Feldman, 2005; Mortimer, 2000; Olszewski, 1996)

 2. **Level II—moderate level of evidence**

   a) Elevation of affected areas may help to reduce swelling with new-onset lymphedema.

   b) Elevation of affected area may improve comfort for patients who are bedridden.

 3. **Level III—low level of evidence**

   a) Provide analgesic support ($) for pain symptoms. (See Pain.)

   b) Bandages ($–$$) may be needed to cover areas where lymphatic fluid is oozing through the skin.

C. Death is imminent.

  Level III—low level of evidence

 1. The goal is to maximize patient comfort.

 2. Application of compression garments, bandages, or massage should be determined on an individual patient basis.

 3. No long-term benefits are available for the patient, and continuation of treatment may increase discomfort. However, treatment of lymphedema-related infection may improve comfort.

Patient and Family Outcomes

A. Patient outcomes

 1. Lymphedema volume is controlled optimally.

2. Optimal physical comfort is maintained.
3. Optimal psychological comfort is provided.

B. Family outcomes
1. Family members have an optimal understanding of their role in assisting with lymphedema self-care activities.
2. Loved ones and caregivers have an optimal understanding of when to contact clinicians (e.g., signs of infection or increased swelling).

References

Armer, J.M. (2005). The problem of post-breast cancer lymphedema: Impact and measurement issues. *Cancer Investigation, 1,* 71–77.

Armer, J.M., & Ridner, S.H. (2007). Lymphedema. In K.K. Kuebler, D.E. Heidrich, & P. Esper (Eds.), *Palliative and end-of-life care: Clinical practice guidelines* (2nd ed., pp. 417–430). St. Louis, MO: Elsevier Saunders.

Badger, C., Peacock, J., & Mortimer, P. (2000). A randomized, controlled, parallel-group clinical trial comparing multilayer bandaging followed by hosiery versus hosiery alone in the treatment of patients with lymphedema of the limb. *Cancer, 88,* 2832–2837.

Browse, N., Burnand, K.G., & Mortimer, P.S. (2003). *Diseases of the lymphatics.* London: Arnold.

Feldman, J.L. (2005). The challenge of infection in lymphedema. *National Lymphedema Network, LymphLink, 17*(4), 1–3.

Finlay, I. (1999). End-of-life care in patients dying of gynecologic cancer. *Hematology/Oncology Clinics of North America, 13,* 77–108.

Guyton, A.C., & Hall, J.E. (2006). *Textbook of medical physiology* (11th ed.). Philadelphia: Saunders.

Hamner, J.B., & Fleming, M.D. (2007). Lymphedema therapy reduces the volume of edema and pain in patients with breast cancer. *Annals of Surgical Oncology, 14,* 1904–1908.

Hinrichs, C.S., Gibbs, J.F., Driscoll, D., Kepner, J.L., Wilkinson, N.W., Edge, S.B., et al. (2004). The effectiveness of complete decongestive physiotherapy for the treatment of lymphedema following groin dissection for melanoma. *Journal of Surgical Oncology, 85,* 187–192.

McNeely, M.L., Magee, D.J., Lees, A.W., Bagnall, K.M., Haykowsky, M., & Hanson, J. (2004). The addition of manual lymph drainage to compression therapy for breast cancer-related lymphedema: A randomized controlled trial. *Breast Cancer Research and Treatment, 86,* 95–106.

Megens, A.M., Harris, S.R., Kim-Sing, C., & McKenzie, D.C. (2001). Measurement of upper extremity volume in women after axillary dissection for breast cancer. *Archives of Physical Medicine and Rehabilitation, 82,* 1639–1644.

Mortimer, P. (2000). Acute inflammatory episodes. In R. Twycross, K. Jenns, & J. Todd (Eds.), *Lymphoedema* (pp. 130–139). Abingdon, England: Radcliffe Medical Press.

Olszewski, W.L. (1996). Inflammatory changes of skin in lymphedema of extremities and efficacy of benzathine penicillin administration. *National Lymphedema Network, LymphLink, 8*(4), 1–2.

Petrek, J.A., Pressman, P.I., & Smith, R.A. (2000). Lymphedema: Current issues in research and management. *CA: A Cancer Journal for Clinicians, 50,* 292–307.

Ridner, S.H. (2002). Breast cancer lymphedema: Pathophysiology and risk reduction guidelines. *Oncology Nursing Forum, 29,* 1285–1293.

Ridner, S.H., Montgomery, L.D., Hepworth, J.T., Stewart, B.R., & Armer, J.M. (2007). Comparison of upper limb volume measurement techniques and arm symptoms between healthy volunteers and individuals with known lymphedema. *Lymphology, 40,* 35–46.

Rockson, S.G. (2001). Lymphedema. *American Journal of Medicine, 110,* 288–295.

Twycross, R. (2000). Drug treatment of lymphoedema. In R. Twycross, K. Jenns, & J. Todd (Eds.), *Lymphoedema* (pp. 244–270). Abingdon, England: Radcliffe Medical Press.

Wilburn, O., Wilburn, P., & Rockson, S.G. (2006). A pilot, prospective evaluation of a novel alternative for maintenance therapy of breast cancer-associated lymphedema [Electronic version]. *BMC Cancer, 6,* 84.

Williams, A.F., Franks, P.J., & Moffatt, C.J. (2005). Lymphoedema: Estimating the size of the problem. *Palliative Medicine, 19,* 300–313.

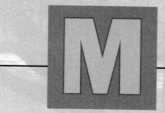

Mucositis

Mucositis

LaDonna Hinkle, RN, MSN, OCN®

Definition

Mucositis is an inflammatory response of the oral, esophageal, and gastrointestinal mucosa resulting in erythema potentially progressing to ulceration (Cawley & Benson, 2005; Harris & Knobf, 2004). It is commonly seen in patients receiving chemotherapy and oropharyngeal radiation (Silverman, 2007). Mucositis is a reaction to dose-limiting chemotherapy and radiation toxicities (Rubenstein et al., 2004).

Pathophysiology and Etiology

Mucositis is a complex multiphase biologic process with a duration of approximately 21 days (Cawley & Benson, 2005; Dodd, 2004). Five phases of mucositis have been identified as initiation, up-regulation and message generation, signaling and amplification, ulceration, and healing (Sonis et al., 2004). Table 28-1 identifies the specific pathophysiologic aspects of these five phases.

Manifestations

- Pain
- Erythema
- Ulceration
- Infection
- Dysphagia
- Anorexia and cachexia
- Weight loss
- Bleeding
- Taste alterations
- Difficult verbal communication

(Dodd, 2004; Harris & Knobf, 2004; Silverman, 2007; Stone, Fliedner, & Smiet, 2005)

Table 28-1. Pathophysiologic Aspects of the Five Mucositis Phases

Phase	Physiologic Reaction	Duration
I—Initiation	Reactive oxygen species are generated by chemotherapy or radiation therapy, leading to DNA damage and cell death.	0–2 days
II—Up-regulation and message generation	Multiple inflammatory cytokines are released, causing thinning of the mucosa and erythema.	2–3 days
III—Signaling and amplification	Further damage to epithelial cells occurs through cytokines, especially tumor necrosis factor-alpha. Cytokines create a feedback loop, amplifying mucosal damage.	2–10 days
IV—Ulceration	As mucosa becomes further damaged, ulcers appear. Pain may be debilitating, and patient is at most risk for infection.	10–15 days
V—Healing	New epithelium develops, and normal oral bacteria are restored.	14–21 days

Note. Based on information from Cawley & Benson, 2005; Sonis et al., 2004.

Management

Management of mucositis should focus on symptom relief and promotion of healing (Dahlin, 2004).

A. Death is not imminent.
1. **Level I—high level of evidence**
   Nonopioid or opioid (oral or parenteral) analgesics ($–$$) (See Pain.) (Scully, Sonis, & Diz, 2006)
2. **Level II—moderate level of evidence**
   (Chung, Hamilton, & Brockstein, 2006; Clarkson, Worthington, & Eden, 2007; DeConno, Sbanotto, Ripamonti, & Ventafridda, 2004; Harris, Eilers, Cashavelly, Maxwell, & Harriman, 2007; Mucositis Study Group, 2005; Scully et al., 2006; Shih, Miaskowski, Dodd, Stotts, & MacPhail, 2002; Stricker & Sullivan, 2003)
   a) Basic oral care
      (1) Brush teeth with soft toothbrush twice daily.
      (2) Floss daily (only if the patient's platelet count is greater than 50,000).
      (3) Use bland rinses four times a day (see below).
      (4) Apply nonpetroleum lip moisturizer.
   b) Anti-inflammatory and pain reduction agents
      (1) Multiagent ("Magic") mouthwash ($)

(2) Tetracaine ($)
   c) Biologic response modifiers
      (1) Granulocyte–colony-stimulating factor: Filgrastim (Neupogen®) ($$$)—3 mcg/kg subcutaneous (SC) during radiation therapy
      (2) Granulocyte macrophage–colony-stimulating factor: Sargramostim (Leukine®) ($$$)—5 mcg/kg SC for five days
      (3) Immunoglobulin ($$$)—10 ml intramuscular day one, 5 ml day two, 5 ml day four.
      (4) Flurbiprofen tooth patch ($$)—15 mg applied to a natural tooth
   d) Cytoprotective agents
      (1) Amifostine (Ethyol®) ($$$)—Optimal dose is not established.
      (2) Benzydamine HCl—15 ml po. Rinse for two minutes, four to eight times daily (not available in the United States)
      (3) Glutamine (L-glutamine) ($)—2 g in 30 ml 0.9 normal saline solution po. Rinse four times daily.
   e) Other
      (1) Allopurinol (Zyloprim®) mouth rinse ($)—300 mg dissolved in water. Rinse for one minute four to six times daily.
      (2) Low-level laser therapy ($$$)
      (3) Zinc sulfate ($)—Optimal dose is not established.
3. **Level III—low level of evidence**
   (Chung et al., 2006; Hsu, Toljanic, Bedard, & Joyce, 2006; McGuire, Correa, Johnson, & Wienandts, 2006; Stricker & Sullivan, 2003)
   a) Use bland rinses (e.g., sterile water, normal saline, sodium bicarbonate, salt and baking soda) ($) four times a day.
   b) Encourage the patient to avoid tobacco and alcohol.
   c) Avoid offering acidic, spicy, and salty foods.
   d) Treat infection with an appropriate antimicrobial or antifungal agent.
   e) Maintain adequate hydration.

B. Death is imminent.
   1. Priority at this time should focus on maintaining the patient's comfort.
   2. Use opioids for pain, and provide basic oral care as needed.

Patient Outcomes

A. Obtain optimal relief from pain and dysphagia.

B. Maintain optimal nutrition and fluid intake.

References

Cawley, M.M., & Benson, L.M. (2005). Current trends in managing oral mucositis. *Clinical Journal of Oncology Nursing, 9,* 584–592.

Chung, T., Hamilton, R., & Brockstein, B. (2006). *Complications of radiotherapy for head and neck cancer.* Retrieved May 16, 2007, from http://www.uptodateonline.com

Clarkson, J.E., Worthington, H.V., & Eden, O.B. (2007). Interventions for treating oral mucositis for patients with cancer receiving treatment. *Cochrane Database of Systematic Reviews 2002*, Issue 1. Art. No.: CD001973. DOI: 10.1002/14651858.CD001973.pub3

Dahlin, C. (2004). Oral complications at the end of life. *American Journal of Nursing, 104*(7), 40–47.

DeConno, F., Sbanotto, A., Ripamonti, C., & Ventafridda, V. (2004). Mouthcare. In D. Doyle, G. Hanks, N. Cherny, & K. Calman (Eds.), *Oxford textbook of palliative medicine* (3rd ed., pp. 673–687). New York: Oxford University Press.

Dodd, M. (2004). The pathogenesis and characterization of oral mucositis associated with cancer therapy. *Oncology Nursing Forum, 31*(Suppl. 4), 5–11.

Harris, D., Eilers, J., Cashavelly, B., Maxwell, C., & Harriman, A. (2007). *ONS Putting Evidence Into Practice: Mucositis: What interventions are effective for managing oral mucositis in people receiving treatment for cancer?* [Brochure]. Pittsburgh, PA: Oncology Nursing Society.

Harris, D.J., & Knobf, M.T. (2004). Assessing and managing chemotherapy-induced mucositis pain. *Clinical Journal of Oncology Nursing, 8,* 622–628.

Hsu, K., Toljanic, J., Bedard, J., & Joyce, R. (2006). *Oral toxicity associated with chemotherapy*. Retrieved May 16, 2007, from http://www.uptodateonline.com

McGuire, D.B., Correa, M.E., Johnson, J., & Weinandts, P. (2006). The role of basic oral care and good clinical practice principles in the management of oral mucositis. *Supportive Care in Cancer, 14,* 541–547.

Mucositis Study Group. (2005). *Summary of evidence-based clinical practice guidelines for care of patients with oral and gastrointestinal mucositis*. Retrieved April 15, 2007, from http://www.mascc .org/media/Resource_centers/Guidelines_table_12_Oct_05.doc

Rubenstein, E.B., Petereson, D.E., Schubert, M., Keefe, D., McGuire, D., Epstein, J., et al. (2004). Clinical practice guidelines for the prevention and treatment of cancer therapy-induced oral and gastrointestinal mucositis. *Cancer, 100*(Suppl. 9), 2026–2046.

Scully, C., Sonis, S., & Diz, P.D. (2006). Oral mucositis. *Oral Diseases, 12,* 229–241.

Shih, A., Miaskowski, C., Dodd, M.J., Stotts, N.A., & MacPhail, L. (2002). A research review of the current treatments for radiation-induced oral mucositis in patients with head and neck cancer. *Oncology Nursing Forum, 29,* 1063–1080.

Silverman, S., Jr. (2007). Diagnosis and management of oral mucositis. *Journal of Supportive Oncology, 5*(Suppl. 1), 13–21.

Sonis, S.T., Elting, L.S., Keefe, D., Peterson, D.E., Schubert, M., Hauer-Jensen, M., et al. (2004). Perspectives on cancer therapy-induced mucosal injury: Pathogenesis, measurement, epidemiology, and consequences for patients. *Cancer, 100*(Suppl. 9), 1995–2025.

Stone, R., Fliedner, M.C., & Smiet, A.C. (2005). Management of oral mucositis in patients with cancer. *European Journal of Oncology Nursing, 9*(Suppl. 1), S24–S32.

Stricker, C.T., & Sullivan, J. (2003). Evidence-based oncology oral care clinical practice guidelines: Development, implementation, and evaluation. *Clinical Journal of Oncology Nursing, 7,* 222–227.

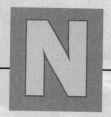

Nausea and Vomiting

Nausea and Vomiting

Mellar P. Davis, MD, FCCP

Definitions

Nausea is an unpleasant sensation of the need to vomit often associated with diaphoresis, lightheadedness, and pallor. *Retching* is the spasmodic movement of the diaphragm and abdominal muscles without retroperistalsis. *Vomiting* results from diaphragmatic intercostal and abdominal muscle contraction, lower esophageal and pyloric relaxation, followed by retroperistalsis (Davis & Walsh, 2000; Twycross & Back, 1998).

Pathophysiology and Etiology

Nausea and vomiting are common symptoms, reported in 40%–70% of patients with advanced cancer (Komurcu, Nelson, & Walsh, 2001; Mannix, 2006; Stephenson & Davies, 2006). Patients can have isolated nausea, isolated vomiting, or the combination of nausea and vomiting (Twycross & Back, 1998). Serious complications result from uncontrolled nausea and vomiting, including dehydration, electrolyte disturbance, and malnutrition. Unresolved nausea can be demoralizing and significantly reduces quality of life. Nausea and vomiting can worsen other symptoms associated with cancer, including anorexia, pain, and fatigue (Davis & Walsh, 2000). The causes of nausea and vomiting in advanced cancer unrelated to chemotherapy have been classified prospectively in three studies and are listed in Table 29-1 (Bentley & Boyd, 2001; Lichter, 1993; Stephenson & Davies).

Chemical etiologies include opioids, anticonvulsants, antibiotics, antidepressants, uremia, hepatic encephalopathy, hypercalcemia, hyponatremia, and ketoacidosis. Impaired gastric emptying and gastric stasis may be caused by drugs (opioids, anticholinergics, tricyclic antidepressants, phenothiazine), or because of paraneoplastic autonomic failure, a "squashed" stomach caused by ascites, hepatomegaly, or splenomegaly. Gastric outlet obstruction occurs from intra- or extraluminal tumor metastases. Visceral and serosal causes involve peritoneal carcinomatosis, intestinal obstruction, mesenteric metastasis, retroperitoneal tumor, gastroenteritis, abdominal radiation, or constipation with impaction. Cranial causes originate from leptomeningeal metastasis, brain stem or posterior fossa metastasis,

Table 29-1. Specific Causes of Nausea and Vomiting	
Reference	**Causes**
Lichter, 1993	Chemical Visceral Central nervous system Vestibular
Bentley & Boyd, 2001	Chemical or metabolic Gastric stasis or obstruction Regurgitant or intestinal Obstruction Unclear or multiple causes
Stephenson & Davies, 2006	Chemical Gastric stasis Visceral or cranial Vestibular or cortical

or increased intracranial pressure. Vestibular causes for nausea and vomiting involve drug toxicity (opioids), motion sickness, labyrinthitis, or base-of-skull metastasis. Cortical etiologies are principally anxiety or uncontrolled pain (Bentley & Boyd, 2001; Lichter, 1993; Stephenson & Davies, 2006).

Clinicians are able to determine a clear etiology in 75% of patients, whereas 25% of individuals will have obscure origins. Ideas about etiology change with further evaluation (Stephenson & Davies, 2006). Approximately 50% of patients will have a reversible cause of nausea and vomiting (Bentley & Boyd, 2001). Half of patients have nausea and vomiting for greater than two weeks prior to evaluation (Stephenson & Davies). Nearly 25% of patients have two or more different causes of nausea and vomiting (Stephenson & Davies).

Manifestations
Symptom History

The key features to chemical- or metabolic-type nausea and vomiting in contrast to gastric stasis or outlet obstruction are the presence of severe persistent nausea and ineffective retching (Bentley & Boyd, 2001). Nausea usually is rated by the patient as severe. Patients with gastric stasis or outlet obstruction have intermittent nausea that is moderate in severity and relieved with vomiting (Bentley & Boyd). Colic and the inability to pass stool are helpful associated findings. Early satiety, headaches, hiccups, reflux, and the type or amount of vomitus are not useful information when allocating a cause for nausea and vomiting (Bentley & Boyd).

Physical Findings

Specific physical findings will help in identifying the etiology of nausea and vomiting. Clinical manifestations suggestive of nausea and vomiting etiology include the following (Davis & Walsh, 2000).

- Papilledema
- Focal or multifocal neurologic deficits
- Stomatitis
- Hepatomegaly
- Splenomegaly
- Ascites
- Succussion splash
- High-pitched bowel sounds or borborygmi
- Periumbilical nodes (Sister Mary Joseph nodes)
- Rectal impaction
- Blumer shelf on rectal examination

Laboratory examination can be helpful in determining the degree of dehydration and detecting hypercalcemia, hyponatremia, uremia, and hyperglycemia, which may cause nausea and vomiting. A flat plate abdominal radiograph can screen for obstipation and intestinal obstruction.

Management

A. General measures: Two approaches have demonstrated evidence of benefit in managing nausea and vomiting in advanced cancer (Glare, Pereira, Kristjanson, Stockler, & Tattersall, 2004; Lichter, 1993; Stephenson & Davies, 2006).
   1. Treatment based upon clinically determined etiology
      a) The etiologic approach to management uses guidelines based upon cause and presumed neurotransmitters involved in generating nausea and vomiting.
      b) Cause is determined by the pattern of nausea and vomiting, associated symptoms (e.g., abdominal pain, constipation, headache), and results from radiographs.
      c) Response rates are determined for the entire guideline and not for individual drugs.
      d) The effectiveness of individual drugs cannot be determined in these studies.
   2. Treatment based on an empiric approach
      a) The empiric approach evaluates the evidence for single-drug responses and grades the evidence by the strength of the study (i.e., level I, level II, or level III).
      b) Table 29-2 is a tabulation of single-drug responses and level of evidence for which recommendations can be made.
   3. Etiologic approaches to managing nausea and vomiting have level II evidence for use.
   4. Empiric single-drug trials cannot be compared with trials that use etiologic approaches to management (Glare et al., 2004). Therefore, etiologic- and empiric-based guidelines should not be seen as conflicting recommendations. Table 29-3 lists recommended drug choices based upon etiologic guidelines.

Table 29-2. Level of Evidence by Individual Agent in Controlling Nausea and Vomiting

Drug	Evidence
Metoclopramide	Level I
Corticosteroids	Level I (bowel obstruction)
Serotonin receptor antagonists	Level I (opioid-induced nausea, added to phenothiazine)
Cyclizine	Level II
Corticosteroids	Level II
Olanzapine	Level II
Haloperidol	Level III
Cannabinoids	Level III
Benzodiazepines	Level III

Note. Based on information from Glare et al., 2004.

B. Pharmacologic interventions
   1. Half to two-thirds of patients will require parenteral drug administrations, either by IV or subcutaneous (SC) routes.
   2. Nearly 25% will remain on parenteral antiemetics until death (Stephenson & Davies, 2006).
   3. One-third will require more than one antiemetic to control nausea and vomiting (Stephenson & Davies, 2006).
   4. Bowel obstruction requires ancillary medications that reduce bowel secretions and colic (e.g., hyoscine butylbromide [$], hyoscine hydrobromide [$], glycopyrrolate [$], and/or octreotide [$$$]) with standard antiemetics (e.g., haloperidol [$], levomepromazine [$], cyclizine [$], chlorpromazine [$]) (Ripamonti et al., 2000, 2001).
   5. Corticosteroids (dexamethasone [$]—6–16 mg po/IV/SC per day) can be used to reduce nausea and vomiting symptoms that have not responded well to standard antiemetics (Feuer & Broadley, 1999).
   6. Some medications are not available in the United States but can be substituted with good evidence of efficacy for substitution.
      a) Either chlorpromazine or olanzapine ($$$) can be used instead of levomepromazine because of similar receptor profiles and clinical evidence of effectiveness (Fink & Winslow, 1955; Homburger & Smithy, 1954; Passik et al., 2002; Srivastava, Brito-Dellan, Davis, Leach, & Lagman, 2003).
      b) Glycopyrrolate ($) can be used instead of hyoscine butylbromide.

Table 29-3. Antiemetic Recommendations Based on Etiologic Factors

Emetic Stimulus	Neurotransmitter Receptor	Antiemetic
Chemical or metabolic	D_2	Haloperidol
Gastric stasis	$5HT_4$	Metoclopramide Domperidone
Visceral or serosal	H_1, M	Cyclizine
Cranial	H_1	Cyclizine
Vestibular	M_1, H_1	Hyoscine

Emetic Stimulus	Drug
Chemical or metabolic	Haloperidol Levomepromazine Cyclizine
Gastric stasis or obstruction	Metoclopramide Domperidone
Regurgitant	Metoclopramide Haloperidol Levomepromazine
Intestinal obstruction	Levomepromazine
Visceral or serosal	Domperidone Octreotide Hyoscine butylbromide
Cranial disease	Cyclizine
Unclear or multiple causes	Haloperidol Cyclizine Levomepromazine

Emetic Stimulus	First-Line Drug	Second-Line Drug
Chemical or metabolic	Haloperidol (1.5–6 mg po daily or 3–6 mg IV daily)	Levomepromazine
Gastric stasis or obstruction	Metoclopramide (30–80 mg po daily or 30–60 mg IV daily)	Levomepromazine
Visceral or serosal	Cyclizine (50 mg po daily)	Levomepromazine
Cranial	Cyclizine (50 mg po daily) Dexamethasone (6–16 mg IV/SC/po daily)	Levomepromazine
Vestibular	Cyclizine (50 mg po daily)	Levomepromazine
Cortical (anxiety)	Lorazepam (1–2 mg po/IV every four hours)	Levomepromazine
Indeterminate cause	Levomepromazine (6.25–25 mg po daily)	Empiric

D—dopamine; $5HT_4$—serotonin; H—histaminic; M—muscarinic

Note. Based on information from Bentley & Boyd, 2001; Lichter, 1993; Stephenson & Davies, 2006.

    c) Combinations of medication should be made on a rational basis based upon receptor profiles that are not overlapping if individuals are not responding to single agents.

    d) The addition of a $5HT_3$ receptor antagonist, such as tropisetron ($$$), will improve nausea and vomiting that has failed to respond to phenothiazines (Mystakidou, Befon, Liosisi, & Vlachos, 1998a, 1998b).

C. Nonpharmacologic interventions

  1. Stents ($$$) can be used to treat nausea and vomiting associated with bowel obstruction (Aymaz & Dormann, 2007; Frech & Adler, 2007; Repici et al., 2007).

  2. Percutaneous endoscopic gastrostomy (PEG) drainage tubes ($$) can be used to relieve gastric outlet obstructions or intestinal obstructions unrelieved by medical management in patients who are not surgical candidates (Cannizzaro et al., 1995; Pothuri et al., 2005).

  3. Cranial radiation ($$$) may relieve nausea, vomiting, vertigo, and dysphagia in patients with cerebral metastases, base-of-skull metastases, or leptomeningeal carcinomas as an ancillary treatment with corticosteroids (Hoegler, 1997; Soffietti, Ruda, & Mutani, 2002).

  4. Paracentesis may temporarily relieve nausea associated with ascites (Ross et al., 1989).

  5. Hydration, bisphosphonates ($$$), and/or calcitonin ($$$) can be used to reduce calcium levels from hypercalcemia and to treat nausea caused by elevated calcium levels (Lamy, Jenzer-Closuit, & Burckhardt, 2001; Zojer, Keck, & Pecherstorfer, 1999).

  6. Enemas ($) will relieve fecal impaction and associated nausea.

  7. Stimulation of the P_6 acupuncture point by acupressure ($) or acupuncture ($$) can supplement antiemetics (Ezzo, Streitberger, & Schneider, 2006).

D. Death is not imminent.

  1. Treat reversible causes.

  2. Use pharmacologic interventions.

  3. Use nonpharmacologic interventions such as stents and PEG tubes once the etiology is clarified (Davis & Walsh, 2000).

  4. Treat complications related to nausea and vomiting, such as dehydration and electrolyte abnormalities.

E. Death is imminent.

  1. Nausea will be accompanied by delirium, dysphasia, anorexia, and a rapidly declining performance status near the end of life.

  2. Forty-eight percent of dying patients will suffer from nausea and vomiting (Davis, Frandsen, Dickerson, & Ripamonti, 2002).

  3. Investigations using laboratory testing and radiographs should be avoided for symptom management.

4. Oral medications frequently are not an option because of dysphagia, changing levels of consciousness, and nausea; most patients will require parenteral antiemetics.

5. Optimal empiric management is outlined in Table 29-4.

Table 29-4. Management of Nausea and Vomiting When Death Is Imminent			
Agent	**IV**	**Subcutaneous**	**Per Rectum**
Chlorpromazine	12.5–25 mg	–	25 mg
Prochlorperazine	10–25 mg	–	25 mg
Haloperidol	1–2 mg	1–2 mg	–
Promethazine	25 mg	–	25 mg
Metoclopramide	10 mg	10 mg	10 mg
Olanzapine[a]	–	–	–

[a] 5 mg sublingual every 12 hours.

Note. Based on information from Davis et al., 2002.

Patient Outcomes

A. Nausea and vomiting are relieved.

B. Complications from nausea and vomiting are effectively treated.

C. Oral intake is optimal.

References

Aymaz, S., & Dormann, A.J. (2007). Stents and bowel obstruction: Practical considerations. *Journal of Supportive Oncology, 5,* 322–333.

Bentley, A., & Boyd, K. (2001). Use of clinical pictures in the management of nausea and vomiting: A prospective audit. *Palliative Medicine, 15,* 247–253.

Cannizzaro, R., Bortoluzzi, F., Valentini, M., Scarabelli, C., Campagnutta, E., Sozzi, M., et al. (1995). Percutaneous endoscopic gastrostomy as a decompressive technique in bowel obstruction due to abdominal carcinomatosis. *Endoscopy, 27,* 317–320.

Davis, M., Frandsen, J., Dickerson, E., & Ripamonti, C. (2002). Prescribing for the actively dying patient: Principles and practice. *Journal of Terminal Oncology, 1,* 19–32.

Davis, M.P., & Walsh, D. (2000). Treatment of nausea and vomiting in advanced cancer. *Supportive Care in Cancer, 8,* 444–452.

Ezzo, J., Streitberger, K., & Schneider, A. (2006). Cochrane systematic reviews examine P6 acupuncture point stimulation of nausea and vomiting. *Journal of Alternative and Complementary Medicine, 12,* 489–495.

Feuer, D.J., & Broadley, K.E. (1999). Corticosteroids for the resolution of malignant bowel obstruction in advanced gynaecological and gastrointestinal cancer. *Cochrane Database of Systematic Reviews 1999*, Issue 3. Art. No.: CD001219. DOI: 10.1002/14651858.CD001219.

Fink, S., & Winslow, W.A. (1955). Anti-emetic effect of chlorpromazine (Thorazine) in cancer patients. *Gastroenterology, 28,* 731–735.

Frech, E.J., & Adler, D.G. (2007). Endoscopic therapy for malignant bowel obstruction. *Journal of Supportive Oncology, 5,* 303–310.

Glare, P., Pereira, G., Kristjanson, L.J., Stockler, M., & Tattersall, M. (2004). Systematic review of the efficacy of antiemetics in the treatment of nausea in patients with far-advanced cancer. *Supportive Care in Cancer, 12,* 432–440.

Hoegler, D. (1997). Radiotherapy for palliation of symptoms in incurable cancer. *Current Problems in Cancer, 21,* 129–183.

Homburger, F., & Smithy, G. (1957). Prochlorperazine for the treatment of nausea and vomiting in patients with advanced cancer and other chronic diseases. *New England Journal of Medicine, 256,* 27.

Komurcu, S., Nelson, K.A., & Walsh, D. (2001). The gastrointestinal symptoms of advanced cancer. *Supportive Care in Cancer, 9,* 32–39.

Lamy, O., Jenzer-Closuit, A., & Burckhardt, P. (2001). Hypercalcemia of malignancy: An undiagnosed and undertreated disease. *Journal of Internal Medicine, 250,* 73–79.

Lichter, I. (1993). Results of antiemetic management in terminal illness. *Journal of Palliative Care, 9*(2), 19–21.

Mannix, K. (2006). Palliation of nausea and vomiting in malignancy. *Clinical Medicine, 6,* 144–147.

Mystakidou, K., Befon, S., Liossi, C., & Vlachos, L. (1998a). Comparison of the efficacy and safety of tropisetron, metoclopramide, and chlorpromazine in the treatment of emesis associated with far advanced cancer. *Cancer, 83,* 1214–1223.

Mystakidou, K., Befon, S., Liossi, C., & Vlachos, L. (1998b). Comparison of tropisetron and chlorpromazine combinations in the control of nausea and vomiting of patients with advanced cancer. *Journal of Pain and Symptom Management, 15,* 176–184.

Passik, S.D., Lundberg, J., Kirsh, K.L., Theobald, D., Donaghy, K., Holtsclaw, E., et al. (2002). A pilot exploration of the antiemetic activity of olanzapine for the relief of nausea in patients with advanced cancer and pain. *Journal of Pain and Symptom Management, 23,* 526–532.

Pothuri, B., Montemarano, M., Gerardi, M., Shike, M., Ben-Porat, L., Sabbatini, P., et al. (2005). Percutaneous endoscopic gastrostomy tube placement in patients with malignant bowel obstruction due to ovarian carcinoma. *Gynecologic Oncology, 96,* 330–334.

Repici, A., Adler, D.G., Gibbs, C.M., Malesci, A., Preatoni, P., & Baron, T.H. (2007). Stenting of the proximal colon in patients with malignant large bowel obstruction: Techniques and outcomes. *Gastrointestinal Endoscopy, 66,* 940–944.

Ripamonti, C., Mercadante, S., Groff, L., Zecca, E., DeConno, F., & Casuccio, A. (2000). Role of octreotide, scopolamine butylbromide, and hydration in symptom control of patients with inoperable bowel obstruction and nasogastric tubes: A prospective randomized trial. *Journal of Pain and Symptom Management, 19,* 23–34.

Ripamonti, C., Twycross, R., Baines, M., Bozzetti, F., Capri, S., DeConno, F., et al. (2001). Clinical-practice recommendations for the management of bowel obstruction in patients with end-stage cancer. *Supportive Care in Cancer, 9,* 223–233.

Ross, G.J., Kessler, H.B., Clair, M.R., Gatenby, R.A., Hartz, W.H., & Ross, L.V. (1989). Sonographically guided paracentesis for palliation of symptomatic malignant ascites. *American Journal of Roentgenology, 153,* 1309–1311.

Soffietti, R., Ruda, R., & Mutani, R. (2002). Management of brain metastases. *Journal of Neurology, 249,* 1357–1369.

Srivastava, M., Brito-Dellan, N., Davis, M.P., Leach, M., & Lagman, R. (2003). Olanzapine as an antiemetic in refractory nausea and vomiting in advanced cancer. *Journal of Pain and Symptom Management, 25,* 578–582.

Stephenson, J., & Davies, A. (2006). An assessment of aetiology-based guidelines for the management of nausea and vomiting in patients with advanced cancer. *Supportive Care in Cancer, 14,* 348–353.

Twycross, R., & Back, I. (1998). Nausea and vomiting in advanced cancer. *European Journal of Palliative Care, 5,* 39–45.

Zojer, N., Keck, A.V., & Pecherstorfer, M. (1999). Comparative tolerability of drug therapies for hypercalcemia of malignancy. *Drug Safety, 21,* 389–406.

P

Pain

Palliative Care

Palliative Sedation

Pruritus

Pain

Mellar P. Davis, MD, FCCP

Definition

The International Association for the Study of Pain (IASP) defines *pain* as "an unpleasant sensory and emotional experience associated with actual or potential tissue damage, or described in terms of such damage" (IASP, 1979). Pain may be acute or chronic, transient (intermittent) or continuous, and associated with transient flares of pain (breakthrough pain). An etiologic classification includes nociceptive pain, divided into visceral and somatic, and neuropathic pain (Nekolaichuk, Fainsinger, & Lawlor, 2005; Twycross, 1999).

Pathophysiology and Etiology

The majority (92%) of pain experienced by patients with cancer is related directly to the disease, whereas a small proportion of pain is related to either treatment or associated with comorbidities. Two-thirds of patients with pain suffer from severe pain, and 25% will have more than one distinct pain syndrome. Nociceptive somatic pain occurs in 72% of patients, nociceptive visceral pain in 35% of patients, and neuropathic pain in 40% of patients (Eidelman & Carr, 2006). Table 30-1 outlines the etiologies of pain (Caraceni & Portenoy, 1999).

Manifestations

Neuropathic pain simply is defined as pain in an area of sensory or motor loss. Hence, "positive" (pain) and "negative" (sensory deficits) symptoms occur within the same dermatome from neuropathic pain. Neuropathic pain can be described as numbing, burning, and tingling, either in a "sock-and-glove-like" distribution or along a dermatome (e.g., shingles). Patients may experience allodynia (pain with nonpainful stimulation) or hyperpathia (a hyper response to a usually mild painful stimulus) (Finnerup, Otto, McQuay, Jensen, & Sindrup, 2005).

The author would like to acknowledge Constantino Benedetti, MD, Joshua Cox, PharmD, BCPS, E. Duke Dickerson, MSc, PhD, Peg Esper, MSN, MSA, RN, AOCN®, APRN-BC, Marco Pappagallo, MD, and James Varga, RPh, MBA, for their contributions that remain unchanged from the first edition of this textbook.

Table 30-1. Etiologies of Pain	
Type	**Frequency**
Bone and joint metastases	42%
Visceral infiltration	28%
Soft tissue infiltration	28%
Peripheral nerve injury	28%
Note. Based on information from Caraceni & Portenoy, 1999.	

Nociceptive pain can be inflammatory or noninflammatory and results from ongoing activation of primary afferent neurons. Somatic pain is often localized and described by the patient as being "aching," "squeezing," "stabbing," "throbbing," or "sharp." Transient flares of pain related to activity (termed *incident pain*) are usually associated with severe pain. Pain unrelated to activity *(breakthrough pain)* and pain before the next dose of analgesia *(end-of-dose failure)* are types of transient pain (Caraceni & Portenoy, 1999; Eidelman & Carr, 2006).

Visceral nociceptive pain is not well localized and is often associated with a large affective (emotive) component. Visceral pain is associated with other visceral symptoms (e.g., nausea, colic, urgency, dyspepsia). The stimulation of afferent sensory fibers that follow sympathetic fibers through the thoracic paravertebral ganglion ascend with second order neurons in the dorsal column and are distinctly different from somatic sensory neurons (Drewes et al., 2006). Visceral sensory neurons are highly represented in areas that elicit emotive/affective responses to pain (e.g., insular cortex, prefrontal cortex) and are poorly represented in the sensory cortex that differentiates visceral from somatic pain (Drewes et al.).

Pain Assessment

Pain assessment should include a time frame of the pain experience, location, intensity, radiation, palliative factors, exacerbating factors, and the quality of pain. Identifying what interference pain has made on the patient's physical activity and the degree of distress associated with pain will help to guide the appropriate therapy. Optimal treatment should decrease pain intensity and distress and improve physical function.

Figure 30-1 outlines a helpful mnemonic device, "PQRST." Descriptors provide information about severity, the type of pain, and associated depression.

Visual analog scales, numerical rating scales, and categorical scales (e.g., none, mild, moderate, severe) are used when assessing the pain's intensity and to effectively evaluate the patient's response to treatment. A two-point decrease in a patient-rated numerical pain score (0 represents no pain and 10 represents severe pain) is clinically significant (Farrar, Berlin, & Strom, 2003).

Figure 30-1. Using the PQRST Mnemonic for Pain Evaluation
Palliative factors: "What makes your pain feel better?" Provocative factors: "What worsens your pain?" Quality: "What is the characteristic of the pain? How would you describe your pain?" Radiation: "Does your pain move around?" Severity: "How severe or intense is your pain?" Temporal: "Does your pain change during the day, with treatment, or with movement?"

Management
Pharmacologic Interventions

Most cancer pain responds to oral analgesics and adjuvants. The World Health Organization (WHO) three-step analgesic ladder provides a framework of principles that, when used, leads to pain relief in most patients (Hanks et al., 2001). The most important part of the WHO analgesic ladder is the efficient use of opioids for moderate and severe pain. Treatment is based on pain intensity and progresses from nonopioid analgesics (e.g., nonsteroidal anti-inflammatory drugs [$] or other adjuvants [$–$$]), to weak opioids (e.g., codeine [$], tramadol [$$]), and to strong opioids (e.g., morphine [$], fentanyl [$$$$], oxycodone [$–$$], hydromorphone [$$], methadone [$]). The management of pain by the WHO analgesic ladder has been prospectively validated with a moderate level of evidence (II) and works regardless of pain etiology (Eisenberg, McNicol, & Carr, 2007; Grond et al., 1999; Ventafridda, Saita, Ripamonti, & De Conno, 1985; Zech, Grond, Lynch, Hertel, & Lehmann, 1995). A moderate level of evidence (II) exists for use of fentanyl, hydromorphone, methadone, morphine, and oxycodone in the treatment of moderate to severe cancer pain with a low level of evidence (III) (expert opinion) for morphine as the first opioid of choice (Hanks et al., 2001; Quigley, 2007; Zeppetella & Ribeiro, 2007). Morphine is the first opioid of choice because no other studies to date have found other potent opioids superior. Recommendations for pain management and the level of evidence are outlined in Table 30-2.

Adjuvant analgesics effectively improve pain in patients who have inadequate responses to morphine. Adjuvants are also morphine sparing, allowing for a 30% reduction in the total opioid dose. Antidepressants, anticonvulsants, and nonsteroidal anti-inflammatory drugs improve cancer pain and potentiate opioid analgesia (Gilron et al., 2005; Wiffen, Edwards, Barden, & McQuay, 2007). Laxatives should be used proactively to reduce or prevent opioid-induced constipation (level II evidence) (Miles, Fellowes, Goodman, & Wilkinson, 2007).

Bone metastasis will respond to radiation, surgery, bisphosphonates, or a combination in the majority of patients (Wong & Wiffen, 2007). Single-fraction radiation is as effective as multifraction radiation in relieving pain (level I evidence) (Wu, Wong, Johnston, Bezjak, & Whelan, 2003). Converting morphine to epidural, subarachnoid, or intracerebroventricular administration improves the therapeutic index of morphine predominantly by reducing opioid side effects associated from systemic morphine (level II evidence) (Ballantyne & Carwood, 2007; Kedlaya, Reynolds, &

Table 30-2. Level of Evidence for Pain Management Strategies

Recommendations	Strength of Evidence
The regular dose of morphine should be increased if pain returns before the next dose. Short-acting morphine is given every four hours, long-acting every 12–24 hours.	Level I
No pharmaceutically important differences exist among 12-hour morphine preparations (long-acting opioids).	Level I
Oral/transmucosal fentanyl is effective for breakthrough pain.	Level I
Opioid rotation or route conversion (spinal) will be necessary in patients with inadequate pain control and limiting opioid side effects (e.g., myoclonus, confusion, hallucinations, nausea, vomiting).	Level II
Buccal, sublingual, and nebulized morphine are not preferred because of lack of absorption.	Level II
Oral morphine is converted to subcutaneous (SC) or IV using a potency ratio of 1 to 3 (parenteral to oral).	Level II
SC morphine is preferred over intramuscular morphine because of pain with administration.	Level III
SC morphine is preferred. However, if a central line is available or the patient has generalized edema, erythema, soreness or pain at the SC site, coagulation disorder, or poor peripheral circulation, IV administration is preferred.	Level III
Long-acting morphine dosage should not be changed more frequently than every 48 hours.	Level III
Oral administration of morphine is the optimal route. Both short-acting for titration and long-acting for maintenance should be used.	Level III
Breakthrough dose and titration dose is the same as the four-times-a-day morphine dose.	Level III

Note. Based on information from Hanks et al., 2001.

Waldman, 2002). The addition of spinal bupivicaine, clonidine, or ziconotide will improve pain control when combined with preservative-free spinal morphine (level II evidence) (Stearns et al., 2005). Neurolytic celiac plexus block improves pain associated with pancreatic cancer (level I evidence) (Wong et al., 2004).

Nonpharmacologic Interventions

Nineteen nonpharmacologic interventions for cancer pain have been published (Zaza & Sellick, 1999). These interventions may be used alone or in conjunction with analgesics (Mayer, 1985). The goals of nonpharmacologic interventions are not only to reduce pain and minimize opioid-related side effects but also to improve physical function and self-independence (Doody, Smith, & Webb, 1991). Although several nonpharmacologic therapies exist, the most commonly used modalities are physiotherapy for positioning and maintaining function; heating pads or ice packs to reduce muscle aches, stiffness, or spasm; massage; relaxation and/or distraction therapies; hypnotherapy; transcutaneous electrical nerve stimulation; and acupuncture. Randomized controlled trials have not been done, and most of the evidence is level II or III depending on the modality (Godfrey, 2005).

Patient Outcomes

A. Level of pain is reduced.

B. Function is improved.

C. Minimal side effects are experienced.

D. Quality of life is improved.

References

Ballantyne, J., & Carwood, C. (2007). Comparative efficacy of epidural, subarachnoid, and intracerebroventricular opioids in patients with pain due to cancer. *Cochrane Database of Systematic Reviews 2005*, Issue 1. Art No.: CD005178. DOI: 10.1002/14651858. CD00518.

Caraceni, A., & Portenoy, R. (1999). An international survey of cancer pain characteristics and syndromes. IASP Task Force on Cancer Pain. International Association for the Study of Pain. *Pain, 82*, 263–274.

Doody, S.B., Smith, C., & Webb, J. (1991). Nonpharmacologic interventions for pain management. *Critical Care Nursing Clinics of North America, 3*, 69–75.

Drewes, A.M., Dimcevski, G., Sami, S.A., Funch-Jensen, P., Huynh, K.D., Le Pera, D., et al. (2006). The "human visceral homunculus" to pain evoked in the esophagus, stomach, duodenum and sigmoid colon. *Experimental Brain Research, 174*, 443–452.

Eidelman, A., & Carr, D. (2006). Taxonomy of cancer pain. In O.A. de Leon-Casaola (Ed.), *Cancer pain: Pharmacologic, interventional, and palliative approaches* (pp. 3–12). Philadelphia: Saunders.

Eisenberg, E., McNicol, E., & Carr, D. (2006). Opioids for neuropathic pain. *Cochrane Database of Systematic Reviews 2006*, Issue 3. Art No.: CD006146. DOI: 10.1002/14651858. CD006146.

Farrar, J.T., Berlin, J.A., & Strom, B.L. (2003). Clinically important changes in acute pain outcome measures: A validation study. *Journal of Pain and Symptom Management, 25*, 406–411.

Finnerup, N.B., Otto, M., McQuay, H.J., Jensen, T.S., & Sindrup, S.H. (2005). Algorithm for neuropathic pain treatment: An evidence-based proposal. *Pain, 118*, 289–305.

Gilron, I., Bailey, J.M., Tu, D., Holden, R.R., Weaver, D.F., & Houlden, R.L. (2005). Morphine, gabapentin, or their combination for neuropathic pain. *New England Journal of Medicine, 352*, 1324–1334.

Godfrey, H. (2005). Understanding pain, part 2: Pain management. *British Journal of Nursing, 14*, 904–909.

Grond, S., Radbruch, L., Meuser, T., Sabatowski, R., Loick, G., & Lehmann, K.A. (1999). Assessment and treatment of neuropathic cancer pain following WHO guidelines. *Pain, 79*, 15–20.

Hanks, G.W., de Conno, F., Cherny, N., Hanna, M., Kalso, E., McQuay, H.J., et al. (2001). Morphine and alternative opioids in cancer pain: The EAPC recommendations. *British Journal of Cancer, 84*, 587–593.

International Association for the Study of Pain, Subcommittee on Taxonomy. (1979). Pain terms: A list with definitions and notes on usage. *Pain, 6,* 249.

Kedlaya, D., Reynolds, L., & Waldman, S. (2002). Epidural and intrathecal analgesia for cancer pain. *Best Practice and Research: Clinical Anaesthesiology, 16,* 651–665.

Mayer, D.K. (1985). Nonpharmacologic management of pain in the person with cancer. *Journal of Advanced Nursing, 10,* 325–330.

Miles, C.L., Fellowes, D., Goodman, M.L., & Wilkinson, S. (2007). Laxatives for the management of constipation in palliative care patients. *Cochrane Database of Systematic Reviews 2006,* Issue 4. Art. No.: CD003448. DOI: 10.1002/14651858. CD003448.pub2.

Nekolaichuk, C., Fainsinger, R., & Lawlor, P. (2005). A validation study of a pain classification system for advanced cancer patients using content experts: The Edmonton Classification System for Cancer Pain. *Palliative Medicine, 19,* 466–476.

Quigley, C. (2007). Opioid switching to improve pain relief and drug tolerability. *Cochrane Database of Systematic Reviews 2004,* Issue 3. Art. No: CD004847. DOI: 10.1002/14651858. CD004847.

Stearns, L., Boortz-Marx, R., Du Pen, S., Friehs, G., Gordon, M., Halyard, M., et al. (2005). Intrathecal drug delivery for the management of cancer pain: A multidisciplinary consensus of best clinical practices. *Journal of Supportive Oncology, 3,* 411–412.

Twycross, R. (1999). *Introducing palliative care.* Abingdon, England: Radcliffe Medical Press.

Ventafridda, V., Saita, L., Ripamonti, C., & De Conno, F. (1985). WHO guidelines for the use of analgesics in cancer pain. *International Journal of Tissue Reactions, 7,* 93–96.

Wiffen, P.J., & McQuay, H.J. (2007). Oral morphine for cancer pain. *Cochrane Database of Systematic Reviews 2007,* Issue 4. Art No.: CD003868. DOI: 10.1002/14651858. CD003868.pub2.

Wong, G.Y., Schroeder, D.R., Carns, P.E., Wilson, J.L., Martin, D.P., Kinney, M.O., et al. (2004). Effect of neurolytic celiac plexus block on pain relief, quality of life, and survival in patients with unresectable pancreatic cancer: A randomized controlled trial. *JAMA, 291,* 1092–1099.

Wong, R., & Wiffen, P.J. (2007). Bisphosphonates for the relief of pain secondary to bone metastases. *Cochrane Database of Systematic Reviews 2007,* Issue 4. Art. No.: CD002068. DOI: 10.1002/14651858. CD002068.

Wu, J.S., Wong, R., Johnston, M., Bezjak, A., & Whelan, T. (2003). Meta-analysis of dose-fractionation radiotherapy trials for the palliation of painful bone metastases. *International Journal of Radiation Oncology, Biology, Physics, 55,* 594–605.

Zaza, C., & Sellick, S. (1999). Assessing the impact of evidence-based continuing education on non-pharmacologic management of cancer pain. *Journal of Cancer Education, 14,* 164–167.

Zech, D.F., Grond, S., Lynch, J., Hertel, D., & Lehmann, K.A. (1995). Validation of World Health Organization guidelines for cancer pain relief: A 10-year prospective study. *Pain, 63,* 65–76.

Zeppetella, G., & Ribeiro, M.D.C. (2007). Opioids for the management of breakthrough (episodic) pain in cancer. *Cochrane Database of Systematic Reviews 2007,* Issue 4. Art. No.: CD004311. DOI: 10.1002/14651858. CD004311.pub2.

Palliative Care

James C. Pace, DSN, RN, MDiv, ANP-BC, FAANP,
and Cheri Mann, RN, MSN, MA

Definition, Scope, and Trajectory

Palliative care actively seeks to provide a comprehensive approach for providing relief from discomfort and painful symptoms without curing the underlying disease, thus improving the quality of life for the patient and loved ones. This care is accomplished through knowledgeable and skilled pain and symptom management strategies combined with collaborative efforts to prevent and alleviate suffering and related problems of physical, psychosocial, and spiritual natures (World Health Organization [WHO], 2007). The goal of palliative care is neither to hasten nor postpone death but rather to support quality of life and informed decision making and to facilitate maximum independent functioning. The scope of palliative care extends beyond the limitations (six months) of hospice services, which are aimed at relieving suffering at the end of life. Palliative care includes aggressive and curative measures that precede and differ from what is offered in hospice care (Meyers & Linder, 2003).

Palliative care initially was offered in acute-care hospitals in the early 1900s. The Center to Advance Palliative Care (CAPC) was initiated in 1999 to support the increase and availability of quality palliative care programs across the country. The development of the field of palliative care was spurred by the publication of various seminal studies (Field & Cassel, 1997; Last Acts, 2002; SUPPORT Principal Investigators, 1995) and has advanced significantly in September 2006 when the American Board of Medical Specialties recognized hospice and palliative medicine as an official medical subspecialty. Today, palliative services are offered through consultative teams in hospitals and outpatient settings, through hospice programs, and in transitional homecare settings and are often integrated into intensive care units (Zerwekh, 2006).

When disease and death are viewed along a continuum (see Figure 31-1), palliative care begins with the diagnosis of a life-limiting disease, illness, or condition, which is managed by curative and palliative interventions intended

The authors would like to acknowledge Helen K. McHale, MSN, RN, CHPN, for her contributions that remain unchanged from the first edition of this textbook.

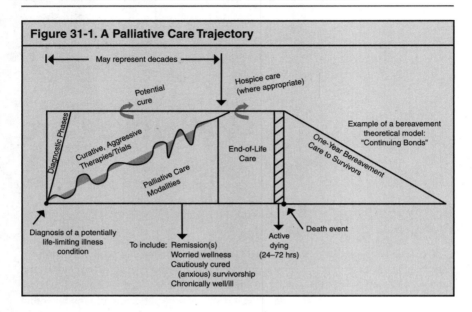

Figure 31-1. A Palliative Care Trajectory

to identify, address, and manage the myriad issues that accompany advanced illness and death.

When interventions are successful in curing or reducing the rate of progressive decline in disease, the patient may choose to disengage from seeking palliative care interventions. In cases where prognosis is poor and curative, aggressive forms of therapies and treatments prove futile, an increase in the intensity of palliative care interventions, such as symptom management and supportive strategies, is heightened and implemented in the patient's plan of care. When appropriate, hospice care referrals may be made as care transitions from curative to comfort when the patient's life expectancy is six months or less. The patient and family are supported through the active dying phase, and survivors are provided with bereavement resources following the patient's death, such as the use of the Continuing Bonds Bereavement Framework (Silverman & Klass, 1996).

Focus of Palliative Care

Palliative care is focused on the patient and family to (WHO, 2007)

- Provide physical comfort, emotional and spiritual support, and relief from distressing symptoms.
- Promote informed, shared healthcare decision making throughout the palliative care trajectory, based on effective communication skills.
- Treat each person as an individual by understanding his or her needs, expectations, and cultural beliefs.
- Utilize the interdisciplinary team across care settings to address the multidimensional needs of the patient and family.
- Enhance the patient's quality of life and positively influence the course of illness.

- Attend to the needs of those who love and care for the dying person.
- Work toward equitable access to palliative care across all ages and patient populations, all diagnostic categories, all healthcare settings, including rural communities, and regardless of race, ethnicity, sexual preference, or ability to pay.
- Commit to the pursuit of excellence and the highest quality of care.

Specific Issues Related to Palliative Care

A. Aging of the U.S. population
   1. As the population ages, the number of chronically ill patients with complex diseases increases. About 77% of all cancers are diagnosed in individuals aged 55 and older (American Cancer Society, 2008). These patients often present with management issues related to social, physical, emotional, and quality-of-life issues.
   2. The rapid increase in medical technology and scientific advances can sometimes outpace providing compassionate, quality care for patients.
   3. Palliative care emphasizes the humane side of health care by refocusing care from the mere preservation of life based on clinical technology to the patients' quality of life based on their preferences and directives (Meyers, 2007).

B. Clinical practice guidelines
   1. The National Consensus Project for Quality Palliative Care (NCP) developed clinical practice guidelines with the aim of improving the delivery of palliative care in the United States (NCP, 2004).
   2. The project responds to the need for uniformly standardized definitions of the essential elements and best practices in palliative care. Although the core elements and focus of palliative care have been previously identified, the NCP defines the eight domains of quality palliative care as follows:
      a) Structure and processes of care
      b) Physical aspects of care
      c) Psychological and psychiatric aspects of care
      d) Social aspects of care
      e) Spiritual, religious, and existential aspects of care
      f) Cultural aspects of care
      g) Care of the imminently dying patient
      h) Ethical and legal aspects of care.

C. Strategies to promote quality palliative care
   1. Provide ongoing assessment and evaluation of pain and symptom management.
   2. Provide effective symptom management through the use of appropriate medications and therapies.
   3. Clarify the patient's advance care directives and healthcare proxy.

4. Encourage the patient and his or her family to actively participate in the planning of advance care plans early in the disease trajectory and prior to disability (Norton & Talerico, 2000).
5. Identify patient and family goals as they relate to palliative and hospice services and help to facilitate the appropriate referrals.
6. Support and guide the ongoing needs of the patient as well as the needs of family and friends.
7. Identify the shift in status from advanced illness management to active dying. The following conditions often distinguish the terminal phase of an illness (Furst & Doyle, 2005). (See Death and Dying.)
   a) Worsening symptoms, especially shortness of breath, fatigue, confusion, discomfort, decreased functional abilities, and pain
   b) Loss of appetite
   c) Weight loss
   d) Increased frequency or severity of exacerbations
   e) Decreased activity and socialization tolerance
   f) Somnolence or insomnia
   g) Increased use of assistive devices
   h) Talk of death
   i) Finishing business
   j) Talking to dead relatives
   k) Withdrawal and unresponsiveness

Patient and Family Outcomes

A. The clinician effectively articulates information regarding diagnosis and prognosis to the patient and family.

B. The patient receives care that reflects continuity, coordination, and comprehension of the palliative care disease trajectory.

C. The patient and family remain informed of expected symptoms and how to manage them effectively.

D. The patient receives customized care based upon personal preferences and available resources (NCP, 2004).

Web Resources and Assessment Tools

- End of Life/Palliative Education Resource Center (EPERC): www.eperc.mcw .edu—A resource for end-of-life and palliative care professionals from the Medical College of Wisconsin. No registration or password needed. Information includes fast facts, clinical guidelines, and links to clinical Web resource centers.
- National Hospice and Palliative Care Organization: www.nhpco.org—A resource for advancing care at the end of life. Content includes communications and

publications, conferences and education, and information regarding palliative care, hospice statistics, and research.

- Regional Palliative Care Program in Edmonton, Alberta, Canada: www.palliative .org—Resources include the Edmonton Symptoms Assessment System and the Edmonton Comfort Assessment Form, as well as links to other useful tools.
- Web site of Dr. Ira Byock, palliative care physician and author: www.dyingwell .com—A resource for defining wellness through the end of life that includes articles, writings, and book reviews.

References

American Cancer Society. (2008). *Cancer facts and figures, 2008.* Retrieved February 25, 2008, from http://www.cancer.org/downloads/STT/2008CAFFfinalsecured.pdf

Field, M., & Cassel, C. (Eds.). (1997). *Approaching death: Improving care at end-of-life.* Washington, DC: Institute of Medicine, National Academies Press.

Furst, C.J., & Doyle, D. (2005). The terminal phase. In D. Doyle, G. Hanks, N. Cherney, & K. Calman (Eds.), *Oxford textbook of palliative medicine* (3rd ed., pp. 1119–1133). New York: Oxford University Press.

Last Acts. (2002, November). *Means to a better end: A report on dying in America today.* Washington, DC: Author.

Meyers, F.J., & Linder, J. (2003). Simultaneous care: Disease treatment and palliative care throughout illness. *Journal of Clinical Oncology, 21,* 1412–1415.

Meyers, S. (2007, May). Care with compassion. *Trustee.* Retrieved June 14, 2007, from http://www.trusteemag.com/trusteemag_app/jsp/articledisplay.jsp?dcrpath=TRUSTEEMAG/Article/data/05MAY2007/0705TRU_FEA_Care&domain=TRUSTEEMAG

National Consensus Project for Quality Palliative Care. (2004). *Clinical practice guidelines for quality palliative care.* Retrieved June 14, 2007, from http://www.nationalconsensusproject.org/Guideline .pdf

Norton, S.A., & Talerico, K.A. (2000). Facilitating end-of-life decision-making: Strategies for communicating and assessing. *Journal of Gerontological Nursing, 26*(9), 6–13.

Silverman, P.R., & Klass, D. (1996). Introduction: What's the problem? In D. Klass, P.R. Silverman, & S.L. Nickman (Eds.), *Continuing bonds: New understandings of grief* (pp. 3–27). Philadelphia: Taylor & Francis.

SUPPORT Principal Investigators. (1995). A controlled trial to improve care for seriously ill hospitalized patients: The Study to Understand Prognoses and Preferences for Outcomes and Risks of Treatments (SUPPORT). *JAMA, 274,* 1591–1598.

World Health Organization. (2007). *Palliative care.* Retrieved December 15, 2007, from http://www .who.int/cancer/palliative/en

Zerwekh, J. (2006). *Nursing care at the end of life: Palliative care for patients and families.* Philadelphia: Davis.

Palliative Sedation

Valarie A. Pompey, MS, APRN-BC, AOCNP®

Definition

Palliative sedation is the use of sedative medication to relieve intolerable, refractory symptoms by reducing consciousness sufficiently enough to improve comfort in a patient with a terminal illness (Levy & Cohen, 2005; Morita, Tsuneto, & Shima, 2002; Muller-Busch, Andres, & Jehser, 2003).

Major tenets for implementation include the following (Bruce, Hendrix, & Gentry, 2006; Levy & Cohen, 2005; Lo & Rubenfeld, 2005).

- Aggressive interventions to relieve symptoms either have been ineffective or resulted in intolerable side effects.
- The goal of sedation is to relieve symptoms and suffering and not to hasten or postpone death.

Specific Issues in Palliative Care

Although at times controversial, palliative sedation is an acceptable intervention to control or alleviate symptoms unresponsive to aggressive traditional treatment modalities. Some of the controversy surrounds the lack of consensus about standards of care and appropriate terminology used to describe the procedure. Other common terms include *terminal sedation, conscious sedation, total sedation, sedation therapy, controlled sedation,* and *sedation for intractable distress in the dying patient* (Bruce et al., 2006; Levy & Cohen, 2005).

The clinician must understand that palliative sedation, physician-assisted suicide (PAS), and euthanasia are not synonymous with each other. Differences lie in the intent or end result.

- *PAS* is defined as "an act that provides a patient with the means and the specific instructions on how to use those means to commit suicide" (Levy & Cohen, 2005, p. 240).
- *Euthanasia* is "deliberate termination of life of a patient by active intervention at the request of the patient in the setting of uncontrolled suffering" (Levy & Cohen, 2005, p. 240).

The author would like to acknowledge Helen K. McHale, MSN, RN, CHPN, for her contributions that remain unchanged from the first edition of this textbook.

Palliative sedation occurs when the palliative care clinician "monitors the delivery of the medication, making adjustments as needed to control distressing symptoms in order to ensure relief of suffering" (Bruce et al., 2006, p. 321).

The outcome or intention of PAS and euthanasia is death; however, the goal of palliative sedation is to relieve suffering without knowingly or intentionally causing harm or hastening death (Bruce et al., 2006; Levy & Cohen, 2005).

Best exemplified with the "principle of double effect" or "doctrine of double effect," four conditions must be met for an act with both positive and negative consequences to be considered morally permissible (Levy & Cohen, 2005; Schwarz, 2004).

- The nature of the act—The treatment is meant to be positive.
- Intention—The clinician's intention is to relieve symptoms with the awareness that hastening of death may be unavoidable.
- The distinction between means and effects—Death is not necessary to relieve the patient's symptoms.
- Proportionality—Relief of refractory symptoms is a compelling reason to put the patient at risk for a hastened death.

The palliative care provider's intention to provide palliative sedation is rooted in the desire to produce a good outcome (relief of suffering), while understanding that the possibility of untoward or unintended side effects (including death) exists (Schwarz, 2004).

Strategies to Promote Use in Palliative Care

Before implementing palliative sedation, discussion that includes the palliative care team, family, patient, and/or proxy should occur. All must be in agreement that previous medical interventions have been unsuccessful and that the symptom is truly refractory. Discussion should include goals of care, common concerns, and clarification of any misunderstandings.

Key Points
- A signed informed consent, with the goals and expectations of sedation clearly and completely disclosed and understood, is placed in the medical record.
- The illness is considered irreversible and terminal, and death is expected, typically in a matter of hours to days.
- The patient has a do-not-resuscitate order.
- A palliative care specialist skilled in the use of palliative sedation has been consulted.
- An independent second opinion has been obtained to support the refractory nature of the symptom causing distress.
- All key points that support the use of palliative sedation, the medication used, dose of medication, and patient response are documented in the medical record.
- Ongoing supportive care is provided to the family, including bereavement programs and support groups (Bruce et al., 2006; Levy & Cohen, 2005; Lo & Rubenfeld, 2005).

The most common symptoms to become intractable or refractory to traditional treatment modalities include (Levy & Cohen, 2005; Muller-Busch et al., 2003; Sykes & Thorns, 2003)
- Pain
- Delirium, anxiety, depression, terminal restlessness, or confusion
- Gastrointestinal symptoms (e.g., nausea, vomiting, bowel obstruction)
- Dyspnea
- Cachexia
- Muscle twitching or myoclonus
- Existential distress or spiritual distress
- Fatigue or malaise
- Bleeding.

Categories and Levels of Sedation

These categories and levels of sedation were developed as a way to unify or clarify terms used to describe duration, levels, and drugs used in palliative sedation (Morita et al., 2002).

A. Degree of sedation
　1. Mild—Consciousness is maintained so that the patient can still communicate with others.
　2. Deep—Almost or complete unconsciousness is achieved.

B. Duration of sedation
　1. Intermittent—Some periods when the patient is alert are allowed.
　2. Continuous—The patient's altered level of consciousness is uninterrupted until death.

C. Pharmacologic properties of medication
　1. Primary sedation—Sedative medications are administered that have not proved to be pharmacologically effective to palliate underlying distress; however, sedation is achieved nonetheless (i.e., benzodiazepines).
　2. Secondary sedation—Reduced consciousness is achieved with medications pharmacologically effective for the palliation of symptoms that are causing underlying distress (i.e., opioids for pain or psychotropics for delirium) (Morita et al., 2002).

Medication Selection and Administration

Selection of medication typically is guided by clinician experience and comfort in using a particular medication, setting (facility versus home), goal of therapy (level of sedation desired), and available route for drug administration. Adjuvant medications may be needed to control specific symptoms not necessarily associated with the identified refractory symptom. Any previously initiated drugs may not be discontinued; however, the dose may need to be adjusted with the addition of palliative sedation. If a pharmacist who specializes in palliative care is available, he or she can assist in drug selection, taking patient demographics, symptoms, and goals of care into consideration.

Midazolam, a benzodiazepine, is the most common drug used for palliative sedation because of its quick onset of action (one to five minutes), short half-life (one to four hours), duration (60–120 minutes), and high therapeutic index (Levy & Cohen, 2005; Lo & Rubenfeld, 2005). The typical loading dose is 0.4–1 mg. A continuous dose range of 0.4–1 mg can be given IV or SC (Levy & Cohen).

Evaluating the Evidence

A. **Level I—high level of evidence**
   1. Because of the ethical and moral concerns associated with performing clinical trials in dying patients, no controlled trials are available to compare the efficacy of medications used for palliative sedation.
   2. Therefore, no treatment exists that has the distinction of having a high level of evidence.

B. **Level II—moderate level of evidence**
   (Levy & Cohen, 2005; Lo & Rubenfeld, 2005; Sykes & Thorns, 2003)
   1. The use of palliative sedation (mostly abroad) has been reported in two retrospective analyses to be 2%–52%, with at least 50% of those patients dying at home achieving symptom control one week prior to death (Bruce et al., 2006; Levy & Cohen, 2005).
   2. Benzodiazepines—This is the most common class of drugs used for continuous sedation.
       a) Midazolam ($–$$)—IV or SC (See the Medication Selection and Administration section within this chapter.)
       b) Alternate drugs used include lorazepam, haloperidol, chlorpromazine, and propofol. ($–$$$)
           (1) Lorazepam—0.5–1 mg every one to two hours in combination with haloperidol.
           (2) Haloperidol—0.5–1 mg every one to two hours for rapid sedation when delirium is the documented symptom needing palliation. However, the effects are very short acting, and patients may experience breakthrough anxiety and extrapyramidal symptoms.
           (3) Chlorpromazine—12.5–50 mg po, IM, or IV every 4–12 hours can be useful when sedation is desired. Side effects, such as hypotension, tardive dyskinesia, and extrapyramidal symptoms, can be of concern with continued use or high doses.
           (4) Propofol—General anesthetic; not recommended unless used in a highly controlled setting and under a physician's direct supervision.
   3. Opioids ($$)—Increasing the patient's opioid dose by 25%–50% may be enough to suppress physical pain that was refractory to nonsedating doses.

However, opioids alone are not as effective as primary sedatives. Doses used also are limited by neurotoxic effects of this class of medications.

4. Neuroleptics ($)—These can be used for routine sedation and are the preferred drug in the setting of agitated delirium.

C. **Level III—low level of evidence**
1. The use of palliative sedation remains controversial. Adding to the trepidation of its implementation is the lack of clinical trials and universally agreed-upon standards of practice.
2. Keeping in mind that the goal of palliative care is to ensure comfort and dignity until the end of life, clinicians should not exclude palliative sedation as a viable option when all other attempts to relieve intractable symptoms have failed.

Patient and Family Outcomes

A. Symptoms are relieved without shortening life.

B. Function is preserved when appropriate.

C. The patient's and loved ones' fears and misconceptions related to the use of palliative sedation are alleviated.

References

Bruce, S., Hendrix, C., & Gentry, J. (2006). Palliative sedation in end-of-life care. *Journal of Hospice and Palliative Nursing, 8,* 320–327.

Levy, M.H., & Cohen, S.D. (2005). Sedation for the relief of refractory symptoms in the imminently dying: A fine intentional line. *Seminars in Oncology, 32,* 237–246.

Lo, B., & Rubenfeld, G. (2005). Palliative sedation in dying patients: "We turn to it when everything else hasn't worked." *JAMA, 294,* 1810–1816.

Morita, T., Tsuneto, S., & Shima, Y. (2002). Definition of sedation for symptom relief: A systematic literature review and a proposal of operational criteria. *Journal of Pain and Symptom Management, 24,* 447–453.

Muller-Busch, H.C., Andres, I., & Jehser, T. (2003). Sedation in palliative care—a critical analysis of 7 years of experience. *BMC Palliative Care, 2*(1), 2.

Schwarz, J.K. (2004). The rule of double effect and its role in facilitating good end-of-life palliative care: A help or a hindrance? *Journal of Hospice and Palliative Nursing, 6,* 125–133.

Sykes, N., & Thorns, A. (2003). The use of opioids and sedatives at the end of life. *Lancet Oncology, 4,* 312–318.

Pruritus

Mary E. Murphy, RN, MS, AOCN®, ACHPN

Definition

Pruritus is defined as an intense cutaneous discomfort occurring with pathologic changes in the skin or body and eliciting vigorous scratching (Pittelkow & Loprinzi, 2004).

Pathophysiology and Etiology

Pruritus is a sensation arising from the activation of cutaneous sensory neural receptors, afferent pathways, and the processing centers. The sensation of itching is transmitted via the C-fibers in the skin to the dorsal horn of the spinal column and the spinothalamic tract of the cerebral cortex for processing, evaluation, and response. Histamine release is a cause of pruritus, but other mediators, such as serotonin, prostaglandins, kinins, proteases, and other physical stimuli, can also cause the disorder (Gomez & Pliczer, 2002). The etiology of pruritus is varied and includes infections; paraneoplastic syndromes; malignancy; and renal, hepatic, hematologic, endocrine, neurologic, autoimmune, skin, medication-induced, and miscellaneous disorders (Butler & Lund, 2007). Additional causes include parasitic infestations, contact induction, allergies, dehydration, and psychogenic disorders (Fazio, 2007). Considerations of the primary diagnoses and any comorbid conditions are essential in determining the cause of pruritus (Lovell & Vender, 2007; von Gunten & Ferris, 2005).

Manifestations

- Itching
- Rash or hives
- Scaling, cracking, or red patches
- Pustules with or without exudates
- Pain

The author would like to acknowledge Peg Esper, MSN, MSA, RN, AOCN®, APRN-BC, for her contribution that remains unchanged from the first edition of this textbook.

- Jaundice
- Burning
- Insomnia
- Fever
- Anxiety
- Erythema
- Sense of crawling on the skin

(Webster, 2005)

Management

A. General measures
1. Identify the source of pruritus (i.e., disease-, medication-, or environment-related).
2. Review the patient's allergy history for severity, onset, location, and dissemination pattern, as well as precipitating factors.
3. Perform a complete physical, appropriate labs, environmental evaluation, psychological review, and extensive review of comorbid conditions and current disease and treatment modalities (Lester, 2006).
4. Rule out dry skin, medication concerns (e.g., allergic responses), hypersensitivity reactions, and infestation, such as scabies and lice, prior to any initiation of therapy (Lester, 2006).
5. Begin treatment with local therapies, such as topical or oral antihistamine therapy, for at least 48 hours before moving to more aggressive therapy (Scot, 2007).
6. General areas of concern for the palliative care patient include hepatobiliary obstruction and cholestatic, uremic, and opioid pruritus (Lester, 2006; Scot, 2007).

B. Death is not imminent.
1. **Level I—high level of evidence**
   Hepatobiliary obstruction (Kichian & Bain, 2004; Pittelkow & Loprinzi, 2004)
   a) Obstruction is caused by interference with the liver's capacity to excrete bilirubin into the biliary system.
   b) Treatment options include inserting a biliary stent and removing the obstruction ($$$).
2. **Level II—moderate level of evidence**
   a) Cholestatic pruritus
   (1) Condition is caused by hepatobiliary flow obstruction (most often related to tumor obstruction).
   (2) Treatment options include the following (Jones & Zylicz, 2005; Kaplan & Chopra, 2007).
   (a) Cholestyramine (Questran®) ($)—4–16 g po daily in divided doses (4 g before or after meals)

    (b) Rifampin (Rifadin®) ($)—150 mg po daily

    (c) Naloxone ($$)—0.4 mg (0.2 mcg/kg/min) IV bolus

    (d) Methyltestosterone (Android®) ($)—10–25 mg po bid

b) Uremic pruritus

    (1) Renal pruritus may occur with chronic renal failure (CRF) and in patients on hemodialysis.

    (2) Treatment options include the following (Germain & Cohen, 2005; Kuypers, Claes, Evenepoel, Maes, & Vanrenterghem, 2004).

        (a) Topical emollients ($)—three to four times a day

        (b) Ultraviolet B (UV-B) therapy ($$$)—three times a week

        (c) Oral antihistamines ($)

            i) Diphenhydramine (Benadryl®)—25–50 mg po every six hours

            ii) Cyproheptadine—2–4 mg po three times a day

            iii) Hydroxyzine—10–100 mg po (syrup), 10 mg/5 mg po capsules four times a day

        (d) Capsaicin ($)—0.025% topical three or four times a day

        (e) Activated charcoal ($)—6 g po daily

        (f) Lidocaine ($$)—100 mg IV during dialysis

        (g) Ondansetron (Zofran®) ($$)—4 mg po bid

        (h) Cholestyramine (Questran) ($)—5 mg po daily

c) Opioid pruritus

    (1) Reaction is caused by the stimulation of the mast cells, which causes cell deregulation and release of histamine.

    (2) Treatment options include the following (Davis & Frandsen, 2005).

        (a) Rotate opioids—Change to fentanyl ($$$), oxycodone ($$), or methadone ($).

        (b) Diphenhydramine (Benadryl) ($)—25–50 mg po every six hours

        (c) Hydroxyzine ($)—10–100 mg po (syrup), 10 mg/5 mg po (capsules) four times a day

        (d) Ondansetron (Zofran) ($$)—4 mg po bid

d) Tumor-related pruritus

    (1) Condition is caused by a release of toxins or cytokines or an auto-immune response.

    (2) Treatment options include the following (Davis & Frandsen, 2005).

        (a) Corticosteroids ($)—IV, SC, or po four times a day (dose based on symptoms)

        (b) Paroxetine (Paxil®) ($$)—10–20 mg po daily

e) Generalized pruritus

    (1) Treatment is based on history and intensity of symptoms.

    (2) Treatment options include the following.

        (a) Antihistamines: Competitive with H_1 or H_2 receptor antagonists

       i) H_1 (first-generation)
- Diphenhydramine (Benadryl) ($)—25–50 mg po every six hours
- Hydroxyzine HCl ($)—2–4 mg po three times a day

      ii) H_1 (second-generation)
- Cetirizine (Zyrtec®) ($)—5–10 mg po daily
- Loratadine (Claritin®) ($)—10 mg po daily

     iii) H_2 (second-generation)
- Cimetidine (Tagamet®) ($)—300 mg po every six hours

(b) Tricyclic antidepressants with antihistamine effect
       i) Doxepin (Sinequan®) ($)—5 mg (maximum dose 150 mg) po daily before bedtime
      ii) Mirtazapine (Remeron®) ($$)—7.5–15 mg po daily before bedtime
     iii) Paroxetine (Paxil) ($$)—10–20 mg po daily

(c) Corticosteroids: Provide anti-inflammatory response
       i) Prednisone ($)—20–40 mg po daily
      ii) Dexamethasone ($)—0.75–2 mg po daily

(d) Local anesthetics: Interfere with the transmission of impulses along the sensory nerve
       i) Lotions with 0.25 or 0.5 menthol ($)—topical three or four times a day
      ii) 2% lidocaine jelly or 5% lidocaine ointment—topical three or four times a day

(e) Topical lotions ($): Provide local cutaneous relief as needed
       i) Sarna®
      ii) Bag Balm®
     iii) Lubriderm®
     iv) Eucerin®
     v) Aveeno®

(f) Ointments to provide cutaneous relief of fungal infections
       i) Nystatin cream or ointment ($)—topical three times a day
      ii) Nystatin and triamcinolone cream or ointment ($)—topical three times a day
     iii) Terbinafine (Lamisil®) spray or cream ($)—topical three times a day

(g) Products to treat scabies or lice infestations
       i) Permethrins ($)—1% cream rinse for lice, 5% lotion for scabies
      ii) Pyrethrins ($)—gel, liquid shampoo for lice

3. **Level III—low level of evidence**
   a) Pharmacologic interventions ($): Emollients to smooth and hydrate skin (Fazio, 2007; Palliative.drugs.com, 2003)
   (1) Aqueous cream 30%, Bag Balm, Balmex®, or vitamin A + D ointment—apply topically four times a day

(2) Colloidal oatmeal cream (Aveeno)
(3) Crotamiton 10% (Eurax®)
(4) Sarna, Eucerin, lidocaine (Lidoderm®)

 b) Nonpharmacologic interventions ($) (Butler & Lund, 2007; Spangnola & Korb, 2004)
  (1) Apply cool/moist compresses.
  (2) Encourage the patient to wear loose clothing (i.e., open-weave cotton blends) and to avoid wearing wool.
  (3) Trim the patient's fingernails.
  (4) Encourage the patient to wear gloves or mitts.
  (5) Instruct the patient to avoid using perfumed lotions and soaps.
  (6) Use distraction techniques.
  (7) Change bed linens frequently and use mild detergents.
  (8) Avoid stressful factors.
  (9) Use moisturizing soaps with neutral pH (e.g., Dove®).
  (10) Increase household humidification.
  (11) Encourage the patient to shower or bathe with tepid water and to avoid using hot water.

C. Death is imminent.
 1. Focus on maintaining comfort through local symptom management interventions that do not require interruption of rest, produce discomfort, or induce untoward side effects.
 2. Administer soothing topical lotions as needed.
 3. Maintain a cool, comfortable environment.
 4. Administer sedation as needed.

Patient Outcomes

A. Pruritus is resolved or is at a level acceptable to the patient.

B. Patient experiences minimal side effects from medications.

C. Skin is free from infection.

D. Additional symptom management concerns are resolved or managed at an acceptable level.

References

Butler, D.F., & Lund, J.J. (2007, March 30). *Pruritus and systemic disease.* Retrieved April 23, 2007, from http://www.emedicine.com/derm/TOPIC946.HTM

Davis, M.P., & Frandsen, J.L. (2005). Cancer pain. In K. Kuebler, M.P. Davis, & C.D. Moore (Eds.), *Palliative practices: An interdisciplinary approach* (pp. 247–267). St. Louis, MO: Elsevier Mosby.

Fazio, S.B. (2007). *Pruritus.* Retrieved April 25, 2007, from http://www.uptodateonline.com

Germain, M., & Cohen, L.M. (2005). Nephrology. In K. Kuebler, M.P. Davis, & C.D. Moore (Eds.), *Palliative practices: An interdisciplinary approach* (pp. 181–196). St. Louis, MO: Elsevier Mosby.

Gomez, D., & Pliczer, J.S. (2002). Dermatologic problems. In B.M. Kinzbrunner, N.J. Weinreb, & J.S. Policzer (Eds.), *20 common problems in end-of-life care* (pp. 203–220). New York: McGraw-Hill.

Jones, E.A., & Zylicz, Z. (2005). Treatment of pruritus caused by cholestasis with opioid antagonists. *Journal of Palliative Medicine, 8,* 1290–1294.

Kaplan, M.M., & Chopra, S. (2007). *Pruritus associated with cholestasis.* Retrieved April 25, 2007, from http://www.uptodateonline.com

Kichian, K., & Bain, V.G. (2004). Jaundice, ascites, and hepatic encephalopathy. In D.H. Doyle, G. Hanks, N.I. Cherny, & K. Calman (Eds.), *Oxford textbook of palliative medicine* (3rd ed., pp. 507–511). New York: Oxford University Press.

Kuypers, D.R., Claes, K., Evenepoel, P., Maes, B., & Vanrenterghem, Y. (2004). A prospective proof of concept study of the efficacy of tacrolimus ointment on uraemic pruritus (UP) in patients on chronic dialysis therapy. *Nephrology, Dialysis, Transplantation, 19,* 1895–1901.

Lester, J. (2006). Pruritus. In D. Camp-Sorrell & R.A. Hawkins (Eds.), *Clinical manual for the oncology advanced practice nurse* (2nd ed., pp. 91–93). Pittsburgh, PA: Oncology Nursing Society.

Lovell, P., & Vender, R.B. (2007, April 9). Management and treatment of pruritus. *Skin Therapy Letter, 12*(1), Retrieved April 20, 2007, from http://www.medscape.com/viewarticle/554692

Palliativedrugs.com (2003). *Skin: Emollients.* Retrieved May 25, 2007, from http://www.palliativedrugs.com/pdi.html

Pittelkow, M.R., & Loprinzi, C.L. (2004). Pruritus and sweating in palliative medicine. In D.H. Doyle, G. Hanks, N.I. Cherny, & K. Calman (Eds.), *Oxford textbook of palliative medicine* (3rd ed., pp. 573–586). New York: Oxford University Press.

Scot, C.L. (2007). Pruritus. In K.K. Kuebler, D.E. Heidrich, & P. Esper (Eds.), *Palliative and end-of-life care: Clinical practice guidelines* (2nd ed., pp. 503–518). St. Louis, MO: Elsevier Saunders.

Spagnola, C., & Korb, J.D. (2004). *Atopic dermatitis.* Retrieved May 15, 2007, from http://www.emedicine.com/ped/topic2567.htm

von Gunten, C., & Ferris, F. (2005). *Fast facts and concepts #037: Pruritus.* Retrieved May 20, 2007, from http://www.eperc.mcw.edu/fastFact/ff_37.htm

Webster, J.S. (2005). Pruritus. In M. Hickey & S. Newton (Eds.), *Telephone triage for oncology nurses* (pp. 185–188). Pittsburgh, PA: Oncology Nursing Society.

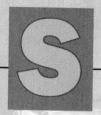

Seizures

Sexuality

Skin Lesions

Seizures

Samuel Gwin Robbins, MSN, RN, MTS, ANP-BC, and
James C. Pace, DSN, RN, MDiv, ANP-BC, FAANP

Definitions

A *seizure* is defined as a recurrent paroxysmal disorder of cerebral function characterized by sudden, brief attacks of altered consciousness, motor activity, or sensory phenomena. Seizures generally are classified by their electroencephalographic features and level of consciousness during an attack. *Simple partial seizures* are associated with a normal level of consciousness and partial motor, sensory, autonomic, or affective symptoms. *Complex* seizures are associated with impaired consciousness and include the following.

- *Petit mal* (absence) seizures are typical in infants and may occur tens to hundreds of times a day. When a seizure begins, the patient stops whatever she or he is doing and assumes a fixed unresponsive stare.
- *Partial complex* seizures combine focal symptoms with an altered state of consciousness. The patient seems awake with fixed or rolling eyes, is immobile, and may repeat words or engage in repetitive behaviors. The patient may become aggressive or hostile.
- *Generalized tonic-clonic (grand mal)* seizures are characterized by sudden loss of consciousness and diffuse muscle rigidity and are followed by myoclonus and muscle fasciculation. At the conclusion of a seizure, in the postictal stage, the patient may move into a deep sleep and complain of headache upon awaking (Simonetti & Caraceni, 2006).
- *Status epilepticus* describes continuous, generalized seizures lasting longer than five minutes, or two or more seizures without full recovery of consciousness between episodes (Caraceni, Martini, & Simonetti, 2005).

Pathophysiology and Etiology

In palliative care, seizures may be caused by primary or metastatic brain malignancy, AIDS, preexisting seizure disorders, metabolic disorders, medications and/

The authors would like to acknowledge Kimberly A. Zielke, MD, for her contribution that remains unchanged from the first edition of this textbook.

or drug toxicities, central nervous system infection, trauma, stroke, hemorrhage, neurologic diseases, or alcohol or drug withdrawal (Simonetti & Caraceni, 2006). Seizures occur when many neurons discharge in an uncontrolled manner, producing paroxysmal behavioral changes (Paice, 2006). Partial complex seizures, which combine impaired consciousness with focal symptoms, are perhaps the most common in palliative care. Witnessing a seizure can be a frightening experience for both clinicians and family members. Evaluation for seizure potential and appropriate planning is required for optimal management (Caraceni et al., 2005). Prophylactic anticonvulsant treatment in patients with brain metastases or primary tumors has not been shown to be of any advantage, nor does it prevent seizure development (Simonetti & Caraceni).

Manifestations

- Alteration in consciousness
- Dramatic change in consciousness coupled with a fall, tonic-clonic convulsions of all extremities, urinary and fecal incontinence, and amnesia
- Some attacks are preceded by an aura; others provide no warning.
- Muscular contractions of a localized area or only one side of the body
- Myoclonic jerking (the twitching or spasm of a muscle or group of muscles)
- Loss of muscle tone

(Caraceni et al., 2005)

Management

A. Death is not imminent.
   Level I—high level evidence
   1. Seizures caused by a primary tumor, by tumor metastasis to the central nervous system, or by a preexisting condition should be treated with anticonvulsants.
      a) Phenytoin (Dilantin®) ($), phenobarbital, or oxcarbazepine (Trileptal®) ($$)—Dosage should be titrated based on individual needs (Caraceni et al., 2005).
      b) Valproic acid (Depakene®) ($$) or gabapentin (Neurontin®) ($$$)—Dosage should be titrated based on individual needs.
   2. For seizures secondary to a metabolic disturbance, such as hyponatremia, hypercalcemia, or hypoglycemia, consider treating the underlying disturbance; medications contributing to these conditions, such as diuretics or hypoglycemics, need to be decreased or discontinued.
   3. Note the patient's drug regimen because medications can induce or lower the patient's threshold for seizures.
      a) All opioids taken at high dosages can cause seizures. Various opioid metabolites have been shown to cause seizures in patients unable to excrete them sufficiently. Therefore, renal function must be closely monitored.

    b) Drug preservatives and additives also can cause seizures.

    c) Medications such as tricyclic antidepressants, phenothiazines, and butyrophenones can lower the seizure threshold.

    d) Abrupt discontinuation of certain drugs, particularly benzodiazepines, barbiturates, and baclofen, can cause seizures (Paice, 2006).

4. All patients at risk for seizures should have medication on hand to be given immediately in the event of a seizure.

    a) Lorazepam (Ativan®) ($) is considered the drug of choice—1–2 mg sublingual, subcutaneous, per rectum, or IV every hour until symptoms subside

    b) Diazepam (Valium®) ($)—5–10 mg per rectum, subcutaneous, or IV every hour until symptoms subside

    c) Midazolam ($$)—30–60 mg subcutaneous or IV every 24 hours (Caraceni et al., 2005)

B. Death is imminent.

Level II—moderate level of evidence

1. Regardless of the cause, the seizure should be treated with a benzodiazepine, such as lorazepam, diazepam, or phenobarbital (Furst & Doyle, 2005).

2. Approximately 10% of patients suffer grand mal seizures as death nears. Providers should manage multifocal myoclonus in order to prevent seizures and the distress they cause a patient's relatives. Should seizures occur, administering subcutaneous midazolam 5–10 mg each hour until symptoms subside or 10–20 mg of rectal diazepam are appropriate interventions. Maintenance doses of an anticonvulsant subsequently should be introduced (Furst & Doyle, 2005).

Patient Outcomes

A. Seizures are prevented, whenever possible.

B. Seizure is rapidly terminated safely.

C. Reversible causes of potential seizure are identified and modified.

References

Caraceni, A., Martini, C., & Simonetti, F. (2005). Neurological problems in advanced cancer. In D. Doyle, G. Hanks, N. Cherny, & K. Calman (Eds.), *Oxford textbook of palliative medicine* (3rd ed., pp. 705–708). New York: Oxford University Press.

Furst, C.J., & Doyle, D. (2005). The terminal phase. In D. Doyle, G. Hanks, N. Cherny, & K. Calman (Eds.), *Oxford textbook of palliative medicine* (3rd ed., pp. 1119–1133). New York: Oxford University Press.

Paice, J. (2006). Neurological disturbances. In B. Ferrell & N. Coyle (Eds.), *Textbook of palliative nursing* (2nd ed., pp. 365–373). New York: Oxford University Press.

Simonetti, F., & Caraceni, A.T. (2006). Seizures. In E. Bruera, I.J. Higginson, C. Ripamonti, & C.F. von Gunten (Eds.), *Textbook of palliative medicine* (pp. 841–848). New York: Oxford University Press.

Sexuality

Blaire Barnes Morriss, MSN, APRN-BC, and
James C. Pace, DSN, RN, MDiv, ANP-BC, FAANP

Definitions

The World Health Organization (WHO) (2002) defines *sexuality* as "a central aspect of being human throughout life [that] encompasses sex, gender identities and roles, sexual orientation, eroticism, pleasure, intimacy, and reproduction. Sexuality is experienced and expressed in thoughts, fantasies, desires, beliefs, attitudes, values, behaviors, practices, roles, and relationships."

Intimacy is defined as a measure of meaning, emotional depth, and love reciprocated between oneself and another. It may include factors such as commitment, attachment, and trust. Intimacy is considered a primary psychological need and is important to individual well-being (Theodore, Duran, Antoni, & Fernandez, 2004).

Specific Issues Related to Palliative Care

Sexuality and intimacy are important to patients and their partners. As chronic disease progresses, sexuality can take on greater meaning, and different forms of sexual expression may be explored (i.e., intimacy). Sexuality and intimacy are a vital link between patients and their partners; therefore, maintaining open lines of communication about sexuality issues throughout the trajectory of illness is beneficial to the relationship. Limited studies have been conducted in examining sexuality in the palliative care setting. Of these studies, most describe a high degree of sexual dysfunction associated with adverse side effects from treatments (Carmack Taylor, Basen-Engquist, Shinn, & Bodurka, 2004; Koseoglu et al., 2005; Walsh, Manuel, & Avis, 2005). Chronic disease can contribute to an altered body image, sexual desire, sexual roles, and partner relationships (Pelusi, 2006).

Despite the need for open and honest discussion regarding sexuality in the face of a life-limiting disease, healthcare professionals tend to either ignore sexuality or feel uncomfortable addressing it (Katz, 2005). Additional reasons for the lack of

The authors would like to acknowledge Beth Cohen, RNC, ARNP, MSN, for her contribution that remains unchanged from the first edition of this textbook.

conversation surrounding sexuality include being unable to find adequate time to engage in these discussions, not knowing how to begin a conversation, and feeling apprehensive about not having enough knowledge to address the patient's questions adequately (Hordern & Currow, 2003).

Clinicians should recognize that patients with chronic disease continue to be "sexual" beings despite living with a poor prognosis. Although the expression of sexuality may become less important as the disease progresses, it often is expressed in different forms (Nusbaum, Hamilton, & Lenahan, 2003). Sexuality can take the form of intimacy and may be expressed through physical touch, as well as expressions of love, warmth, and tenderness (Lamb, 2006). A qualitative study has suggested that patients' emotional connection to others is a key aspect of sexuality, which at times is more important than physical expression alone (Lemieux, Kaiser, Pereira, & Meadows, 2004). Sexuality is an aspect of the need for closeness, touch, pleasure, caring, and play. When sexual activity becomes difficult, impractical, or impossible in chronic debilitating disease or imminent death, expression of affection remains an important way of sharing intimacy.

Manifestations or Complications Related to Sexuality

- Avoidance of intimacy
- Body image concerns
- Depression
- Increased somatic complaints
- Lack of sexual desire
- Inability to achieve orgasm
- Psychosocial difficulty with intimate relationships

(Nusbaum et al., 2003)

Strategies to Facilitate Individual Expressions of Sexuality

A. Death is not imminent.
  1. **Level I—high level of evidence**
     a) Pain resolution (Dunn, 2000; Moynihan, 2007; Nusbaum et al., 2003)
        (1) Pain may be nongenital as a result of disease progression (metastasis) or treatments (antineoplastic and radiotherapy).
        (2) If pain is the primary source of sexual inability, evaluating the origin of the pain is important; if appropriate, discuss pain-reducing strategies, such as implementing analgesics prior to sexual activity.
        (3) Use of opioid or nonopioid analgesics can be determined by the patient's prescriber.
     b) Medications and over-the-counter products (Montague et al., 2005; North American Menopause Society, 2007; Polovich, White, & Kelleher, 2005; van der Laak, de Bie, de Leeuw, de Wilde, & Hanselaar, 2002)
        (1) Erectile dysfunction

(a) Sildenafil (Viagra®) ($$$)—50 mg po 30 minutes to four hours before sexual activity. For geriatric patients and those with hepatic impairment, 25 mg is recommended. Maximum daily dose is 100 mg.

(b) Vardenafil (Levitra®) ($$$)—10 mg po 60 minutes before sexual activity. For geriatric patients and those with hepatic impairment, 5 mg is recommended. It may be taken only once daily.

(2) Vaginal dryness

(a) Estradiol vaginal cream (Estrace®) ($$)—Apply 2–4 g per day for one to two weeks, and then use the lowest possible maintenance dose one to three times per week. Do not use in patients with a history of cancer or cardiovascular disease.

(b) Polycarbophil-based moisturizer (Replens®) ($)—Apply vaginally three times a week or before sexual intimacy. Replens is not recommended for use more than three times a week.

(3) Patient and partner education about the medication should take place prior to being prescribed. The clinician should instruct the patient regarding how and when to take the medication and address any potential untoward side effects and their management.

2. **Level II—moderate level of evidence**

a) Education (Moynihan, 2007; Nusbaum et al., 2003; Stead, 2003)

(1) Provide information about the usual effects of the patient's diagnosis, medications, treatments, and surgery on sexuality.

(2) Discuss high-risk versus low-risk sexual practices in regard to disease transmission (e.g., avoidance of the exchange of blood or body fluids).

(3) Include information on contraception if appropriate.

(4) Inform patients about alternatives to intercourse as an expression of sexuality (e.g., hugging, kissing, massage, caressing).

(5) Discuss conservation of strength, rest periods, and preparation.

b) Positioning (Dunn, 2000; Mueller, 1997; Nusbaum et al., 2003; Steinke, 2000)

(1) Suggest that the patient choose positions that put the least amount of pressure on the painful area.

(2) Instruct the patient to support the painful area with pillows to increase comfort.

(3) For intercourse, recommend a position that allows the patient to be in control of movement and comfort.

c) Counseling and therapy (Dunn, 2000; Onel & Albertsen, 1999; Polovich et al., 2005)

(1) Counseling can occur in a sexual dysfunction clinic, a private practice, or a health clinic.

(2) Costs will vary greatly, as will the number of visits needed.

(3) Exercises may involve the patient learning new skills and techniques and practicing them with a partner.

(4) The clinician should advise the patient to seek counsel from a sex therapist who is a mental health professional (e.g., psychiatrist, social worker, psychologist) or a medical professional (e.g., physician, clinician) specially trained in sexual dysfunction.

(5) Other types of counseling or therapy can be helpful. Issues of depression, body image changes, social changes, and relationship alterations may require supportive counseling.

(6) Support groups can be beneficial and are available in most communities.

3. **Level III—low level of evidence**
   a) Relaxation (Ernst, 2006; Sloman, 2002)
      (1) Patient experience—The patient may be nervous about the length of time since his or her previous sexual encounter and have an altered body image from changes that have occurred from treatments and interventions (e.g., surgical scars, hair loss, weight changes).
      (2) Relaxation techniques—Paced breathing, biofeedback, meditation, massage, visualization, or guided imagery can help the patient to relax and avoid the pain associated with being tense.
   b) Communication (Horden & Currow, 2003; Katz, 2005; Moynihan, 2007; Polovich et al., 2005; Steinke, 2000)
      (1) Open and honest communication should be encouraged to promote healthy intimacy (e.g., patient to partner, patient to clinician, clinician to interdisciplinary team).
      (2) A sexual history of the patient should be performed and considered when establishing the plan of care. The patient may prefer to discuss issues of sexuality with a health professional he or she knows, rather than being referred to a sexual counselor.
         (a) Create a safe space that is amenable to open discussion (e.g., quiet, private, no interruptions).
         (b) Use the PLISSIT model (permission, limited information, specific suggestion, and intensive therapy) in sexual discussions with the patient.
         (c) Use open-ended questions with a nonjudgmental attitude.
         (d) Make no assumptions about the patient's sexuality or relationships.
         (e) Acknowledge cultural and religious diversity. (See Cultural Competence.)
         (f) Lifestyle, gender, sexual orientation, marital status, and age should all be considered when engaging in these discussions.
   c) Addressing barriers to sexuality (Horden & Currow, 2003; Lemieux et al., 2004)
      (1) Address patient-perceived barriers, including lack of privacy, staff intrusion, shared rooms, single beds, and unfamiliar settings.
      (2) Encourage sexuality at home.

(a) Encourage patients to set aside specific times for intimacy and sexuality.

(b) Suggest that patients turn on the answering machine and not answer the telephone or door when they are intimate.

(3) Address sexuality issues in inpatient units.

(a) Promote patient privacy (e.g., a closed door with a "do not disturb" sign during patient intimacy).

(b) If possible, adapt the inpatient environment by keeping lights low and encouraging the possibility of patient intimacy.

B. Death is imminent.

1. Sexuality should be expressed through the patient's level of comfort.

2. Encourage the patient and his or her partner to express intimacy in the form of hand-holding, kissing, eye contact, smiling, or verbalization.

Patient Outcomes

A. Patient and partner are able to identify and discuss sexual problems, dysfunction, or concerns throughout the disease trajectory.

B. Patient is able to discuss sexual concerns and develop strategies with members of the healthcare team.

C. Patient can attain satisfaction with himself or herself as a sexual being.

D. Patient shares intimacy with his or her partner at every possible level.

References

Carmack Taylor, C.L., Basen-Engquist, K., Shinn, E.H., & Bodurka, D.C. (2004). Predictors of sexual functioning in ovarian cancer patients. *Journal of Clinical Oncology, 22,* 881–889.

Dunn, M. (2000). Sexual issues in older adults. *AIDS Patient Care and STDs, 14,* 67–69.

Ernst, E. (2006). *Complementary therapies for cancer.* Retrieved June 18, 2007, from http://www.utdol .com/utd/content/topic.do?topicKey=genl_onc/8402&type=A&selectedTitle=16~27

Hordern, A.J., & Currow, D.C. (2003). A patient-centered approach to sexuality in the face of life-limiting illness. *Medical Journal of Australia, 179*(Suppl. 6), S8–S11.

Katz, A. (2005). The sounds of silence: Sexuality information for cancer patients. *Journal of Clinical Oncology, 23,* 238–241.

Koseoglu, N., Koseoglu, H., Ceylan, E., Cimrin, H., Ozalevli, S., & Esen, A. (2005). Erectile dysfunction prevalence and sexual function status in patients with chronic obstructive pulmonary disease. *Journal of Urology, 174,* 249–252.

Lamb, M.A. (2006). Sexuality. In B.R. Ferrell & N. Coyle. (Eds.), *Textbook of palliative nursing* (2nd ed., pp. 421–428). New York: Oxford University Press.

Lemieux, L., Kaiser, S., Pereira, J., & Meadows, L.M. (2004). Sexuality in palliative care: Patient perspectives. *Palliative Medicine, 18,* 630–637.

Montague, D.K., Jarow, J.P., Broderick, G.A., Dmochowski, R.R., Heaton, J.P., Lue, T.F., et al. (2005). Chapter 1: The management of erectile dysfunction: An AUA update. *Journal of Urology, 174,* 230–239.

Moynihan, T. (2007). *Sexuality in palliative care.* Retrieved March 28, 2007, from http://patients .uptodate.com/topic.asp?file=endoflif/7006

Mueller, I.W. (1997). Common questions about sex and sexuality in elders. *American Journal of Nursing, 97*(7), 61–64.

North American Menopause Society. (2007). The role of local vaginal estrogen for treatment of vaginal atrophy in postmenopausal women: 2007 position statement of the North American Menopause Society. *Menopause, 14,* 357–369.

Nusbaum, M.R., Hamilton, C., & Lenahan, P. (2003). Chronic illness and sexual functioning. *American Family Physician, 67,* 347–354.

Onel, E., & Albertsen, P. (1999). Management of impotence. *Clinical Advisor, 1,* 27–37.

Pelusi, J. (2006). Sexuality and body image: Research on breast cancer survivors documents altered body image and sexuality. *American Journal of Nursing, 106*(3), 32–38.

Polovich, M., White, J.M., & Kelleher, L.O. (Eds.). (2005). *Chemotherapy and biotherapy guidelines and recommendations for practice* (2nd ed.). Pittsburgh, PA: Oncology Nursing Society.

Sloman, R. (2002). Relaxation and imagery for anxiety and depression control in community patients with advanced cancer. *Cancer Nursing, 25,* 432–435.

Stead, M. (2003). Sexual dysfunction after treatment for gynecologic and breast malignancies. *Current Opinion in Obstetrics and Gynecology, 15,* 57–61.

Steinke, E.E. (2000). Sexual counseling after myocardial infarction. *American Journal of Nursing, 100*(12), 38–43.

Theodore, P.S., Duran, R.E., Antoni, M.H., & Fernandez, M.I. (2004). Intimacy and sexual behavior among HIV-positive men-who-have-sex-with-men in primary relationships. *AIDS and Behavior, 8,* 321–333.

van der Laak, J.A., de Bie, L.M., de Leeuw, H., de Wilde, P.C., & Hanselaar, A.G. (2002). The effect of Replens on vaginal cytology in the treatment of postmenopausal atrophy: Cytomorphology versus computerized cytometry. *Journal of Clinical Pathology, 55,* 446–451.

Walsh, S., Manuel, J., & Avis, N. (2005). The impact of breast cancer on younger women's relationships with their partner and children. *Families, Systems and Health, 23,* 80–93.

World Health Organization. (2002). *Gender and reproductive rights.* Retrieved March 28, 2007, from http://who.int/reproductive-health/gender/sexual_health.html#2

Skin Lesions

Doreen A. White, BSN, RN, CWOCN

Definitions

Pressure ulcers are wounds that involve localized injury to the skin and underlying tissue as a result of prolonged pressure or pressure in combination with shear and/or friction (Black et al., 2007). *Malignant cutaneous wounds* are skin lesions that develop when malignant cells infiltrate the epithelium (Fulton, 2006).

Pathophysiology and Etiology

Pressure ulcers are common in the palliative care setting, often as a result of weakness, immobility, and inadequate nutrition (Langemo, Anderson, Hanson, Thompson, & Hunter, 2007). When soft tissue is compressed between a bony prominence and an external surface for an excessive period of time, the blood supply is disrupted, resulting in ischemia, edema, and inflammation, followed by cell death (Pieper, 2007; Sharp & McLaws, 2005). In the dying phase of advanced illness, cachexia or body wasting occurs, and as a result, the skin often "fails" as a consequence of multiorgan failure (Langemo & Brown, 2006).

Malignant cutaneous wounds are caused by abnormal cells penetrating the surrounding lymph nodes and blood circulation, resulting in capillary enlargement with possible rupture. Necrotic tissue may form, and disruption of the lymph vessels can lead to significant drainage. Anaerobic organisms proliferate in necrotic tissue and can create a foul-smelling odor. "The wound is considered fungating once the cancerous tumor penetrates the skin through the processes of ulceration and proliferation" (Schiech, 2002, p. 306). These wounds demonstrate a characteristic fungus or cauliflower appearance (Hospice Pharmacia, 2006).

The author wishes to acknowledge Debra E. Heidrich, MSN, RN, CHPN, AOCN®, for her contributions that remain unchanged from the first edition of this textbook.

Manifestations

Skin ulcers are staged according to their color, size, appearance, and drainage. (Staging systems are described later in this section.) In addition, clinical manifestations may include
- Pain
- Infection
- Anemia
- Odor.

The distress and embarrassment from open, draining, and malodorous wounds can lead to
- Self-concept disturbances
- Disturbance of sleep patterns
- Loss of appetite
- Social isolation
- Anxiety or fear
- Depression.

(Fleck, 2006)

Management

A. General measures: Identify the stage of the lesion.
   1. Pressure ulcers
      a) Suspected deep tissue injury: Characterized by a purple or maroon localized area of discolored, intact skin or a blood-filled blister caused by damage of underlying soft tissue from pressure and/or shear. Presentation may be preceded by painful, firm, and mushy tissue or skin temperature variation (warmer or cooler) when compared to adjacent tissue.
      b) Stage I: Intact skin with nonblanchable redness usually over a bony prominence. Darkly pigmented skin may not have visible blanching; however, its color may differ from the surrounding area.
      c) Stage II: Partial-thickness skin loss presenting as a shallow open ulcer with a red or pink wound bed without slough. Often presents as an intact, open, or ruptured serum-filled blister.
      d) Stage III: Full-thickness tissue loss. Subcutaneous fat may be visible, but bone, tendon, or muscles are not exposed. Slough may be present but does not obscure the depth of tissue loss. Injury may include undermining and tunneling.
      e) Stage IV: Full-thickness tissue loss with exposed bone, tendon, or muscle. Slough or eschar may be present on some parts of the wound bed. This often includes undermining and tunneling.
      f) Unstageable: Full-thickness tissue loss in which the base of the ulcer is covered by slough (yellow, tan, gray, green, or brown) and/or eschar (tan, brown, or black) in the wound bed. Stable, dry, adherent, and intact eschar on heels serves as the body's natural (biologic) cover and should

not be removed (Black et al., 2007; Hess, 2002; Registered Nurses Association of Ontario, 2002).

2. Malignant cutaneous wounds
    a) Stage I: Closed, dry wound that is red or pink in color
    b) Stage I–N: Wound that occasionally opens superficially to drain then closes again. The wound color is red or pink, and drainage may be clear or purulent. These wounds may be painful.
    c) Stage II: Partial-thickness skin loss involving dermal and epidermal tissue. The wound color is red or pink, and drainage may be serosanguineous or sanguineous. These wounds may be painful and tend to be malodorous.
    d) Stage III: Full-thickness skin loss involving subcutaneous tissue. The wound color may be red, pink, or yellow, and drainage is purulent or serosanguineous. These wounds are most likely painful and tend to be malodorous.
    e) Stage IV: Full-thickness skin loss with invasion into deep anatomic tissues and structures. Tunneling is often present. The wound color may be red, pink, or yellow, and drainage is serosanguineous, sanguineous, or purulent. Pain is likely, and the wound tends to be malodorous (Ayello & Schank, 2007).

B. Death is not imminent.
    1. Prevent pressure ulcers.
        a) Keep skin clean and dry.
        b) Prevent friction and shear injuries.
            (1) Use care with patient transfers and when turning the patient, using lift pads, or turning sheets.
            (2) Reduce friction on heels and elbows by using lubricants, thin-film dressings, or protectors.
        c) Encourage mobility and range-of-motion exercises based on the patient's ability to tolerate these activities.
        d) Reduce pressure on tissues.
            (1) Turn and reposition the patient at least every two hours.
            (2) Avoid positioning on trochanter.
            (3) Use supports, such as wedges, pillows, and heel supports.
            (4) Initiate pressure-reducing support surfaces ($$–$$$) for patients at risk for developing pressure ulcers (Pieper, 2007; Wound, Ostomy and Continence Nurses Society, 2003).
            (5) Avoid massage over bony prominences (Registered Nurses Association of Ontario, 2002; Wound, Ostomy and Continence Nurses Society, 2003).
    2. Treat malignant cutaneous wounds.
        a) Use radiation therapy or chemotherapy ($$$) for localized lesions. These treatments may decrease bleeding, drainage, and pain (Fulton, 2006).

    b) Hormonal manipulation ($$–$$$) may be helpful for lesions associated with breast cancer (Moore, 2002).

3. **Level I—high level of evidence**

None

    Clinical practice guidelines can be created based on a review of the evidence available or by consensus, or a combination of both. . . . The government, private foundations, industry, and special interest groups all fund research in wound care, but research that is seeking to change level of evidence may not always be the funding group's priority. . . . We must keep a balance between the need for evidence and the reality of obtaining the evidence. (Edsberg, 2007, p. 9)

4. **Level II—moderate level of evidence**

Wound cleansing

    a) Flush with normal saline using a therapeutic pressure range between 4–15 pounds per square inch (psi).

    b) Using a 19-gauge angiocath with a 35 ml syringe produces an 8 psi pressure stream, which assists in removing adherent material in the wound bed.

    c) A 60 ml piston irrigation syringe with catheter tip delivers a 4.2 psi stream (Registered Nurses Association of Ontario, 2002).

5. **Level III—low level of evidence**

    a) Wound cleansing

        (1) Use of a bulb syringe or a gravity drip through IV tubing will not deliver therapeutic irrigation pressures but may be an alternative for wound cleansing.

        (2) Choose a commercial wound cleanser with a low toxicity index (Registered Nurses Association of Ontario, 2002; Wilson, Mills, Prather, & Dimitrijevich, 2005).

        (3) Malodorous and infected wounds may be managed for short periods using various solutions as listed. Because these solutions are toxic to fibroblasts, they should be rinsed from the wound with normal saline. Concurrent systemic treatment of the infection is usually beneficial (Hospice Pharmacia, 2006).

           (a) Acetic acid solution ($) (equal parts vinegar and water) for *Pseudomonas* infection

           (b) Hydrogen peroxide ($) for mechanical cleansing of crusted exudates

           (c) Povidone iodine ($) for broad-spectrum antimicrobial cleansing

           (d) Sodium hypochlorite ($) (1 part household bleach to 9 parts water) (Dakin's solution) for staphylococcal and streptococcal infections (Ayello & Schank, 2007)

    b) Debridement is the removal of necrotic tissue to decrease infection, reduce inflammation, and increase patient comfort (Ayello & Schank, 2007). The purpose and potential outcomes for debridement should be considered for each individual patient. Fungating tumors manifest persistent necrosis and tumor fragility; therefore, debridement is contraindicated (Fulton, 2006).

(1) Surgical debridement is the most rapid means to remove necrotic tissue but may be unnecessarily painful and require anesthesia (Ayello & Schank, 2007).

(2) Enzymatic debriding agents such as collagenase ($$) (Santyl®) or papain-urea ($$) (Accuzyme®) require a prescription. Follow the manufacturer's instructions for correct application and frequency (Ayello & Schank, 2007).

(3) A product containing papain-urea along with chlorophyllin-copper-sodium complex ($$–$$$) (Panafil®) adds a healing action to the debriding component. This product assists in managing wound odor and promoting healthy granulation tissue (Hess, 2002; Wound, Ostomy and Continence Nurses Society, 2003).

(4) Autolytic debridement uses the body's natural enzymes and leukocytes to remove necrotic tissue (Pieper, 2007). Dressings such as hydrocolloids ($$), semipermeable urethane foam ($$), or hydrogel ($$) promote this process (Ayello & Schank, 2007).

c) Drainage containment

(1) An ideal dressing promotes a moist, but not wet, wound environment.

(2) Shallow, low-draining wounds may be managed with foams ($$) and hydrocolloids ($$). Loosely pack a craterous wound. The dressing must make contact with all the wound surfaces (Hess, 2002).

(3) Deep, highly draining wounds may be packed with alginates, fiber-gelling dressings, or foam wound fillers ($$–$$$) (Pieper, 2007). These interventions provide a moist healing environment, promote autolytic debridement, absorb exudates, and promote comfort (Hess, 2002).

(4) If drainage exceeds 50 ml/day, consider using a wound-drainage collection bag ($$–$$$) to collect exudates, decrease the number of dressing changes required, control odor, and protect surrounding skin (Hess, 2002).

(5) Use of negative pressure wound therapy ($$$) will contain excessive drainage and odor in large wounds but is contraindicated when the wound has a malignant etiology (Gupta et al., 2007; Niezgoda & Mendez-Eastman, 2006).

d) Bleeding control

(1) Choose nonadherent dressings to minimize exacerbation of tumor/wound bleeding.

(2) Apply pressure to visible bleeding vessels if underlying structures can tolerate the pressure.

(3) Apply silver nitrate sticks ($) to pinpoint capillary oozing. Note that this may cause pain, and the patient should be medicated appropriately.

(4) Apply gauze soaked in 1:1,000 epinephrine (Gomez & Policzer, 2001; Hospice Pharmacia, 2006).

(5) Use a coagulant dressing, such as absorbable gelatin ($) (Gelfoam®), oxidized regenerated cellulose ($) (Surgicel®), or QR Powder® ($), to control topical bleeding (Ayello & Schank, 2007; Lagman, Walsh, & Day, 2002; Naylor, 2002).

(6) Consider radiation therapy ($$$) for bleeding in fungating wounds (Ayello & Schank, 2007).

e) Odor control

(1) Apply topical metronidazole ($$$) (MetroGel® gel, 0.75%) (Ayello & Schank, 2007).

(2) Irrigate with parenteral metronidazole solution ($) (Ayello & Schank, 2007).

(3) Place crushed (250 mg) metronidazole tablets ($) into the wound crater. This has been reported to reduce odor and nonsporing anaerobes (Mekrut-Barrows, 2006).

(4) Administer an oral dose of 200 mg of metronidazole twice a day ($) for wound odor; use for limited time because of toxicities of nausea and vomiting (Schiech, 2002).

(5) Administer chlorophyll tablets po.

(6) Use odor-filtering dressings that have a carbon or charcoal layer ($$–$$$) (CarboFlex® Odor-Control Dressing).

(7) Primary dressings devised to manage odor include a hydrocolloid containing cyclodextrin ($$) (Exuderm® OdorShield™) (Fleck, 2006).

(a) Ionized silver dressings ($$) provide a broad-spectrum antimicrobial with anti-inflammatory and healing properties. They are available in transparent films, hydrocolloids, wound gels, and calcium alginates ($$–$$$). Product choice is dependent upon the level of drainage (Queen, Woo, Schultz, & Sibbald, 2005; Warriner & Burrell, 2005).

(b) Deodorizers may mask odors; however, some people may find the scent of the deodorizer offensive.

(c) Dressing deodorizers (Banish®, Hex-On®) may be used sparingly on dressings (Ayello & Schank, 2007).

(d) Commercial room deodorizers, scented candles, or scented oils may be used in the room.

C. Death is imminent.

1. Continue an appropriate positioning and turning schedule to prevent the pain of tissue ischemia.

a) Employ good technique when repositioning the patient, ideally with two people, to prevent discomfort.

b) Evaluate and assess potential discomfort associated with turning and possible tissue ischemia.

     c) Consider analgesic use (short acting) prior to turning and dressing changes.

2. Continue to manage drainage, odor, and pain related to the ulcer.

Patient Outcomes

A. Pressure ulcers are reduced and prevented, whenever possible.

B. Pressure ulcers undergo normal healing process.

C. Infection related to pressure ulcers and malignant skin lesions is prevented, whenever possible.

D. Physical discomfort is relieved, and complications associated with skin lesions are prevented.

References

Ayello, E., & Schank, J. (2007). Ulcerative lesions. In K.K. Kuebler, D.E. Heidrich, & P. Esper (Eds.), *Palliative and end-of-life care: Clinical practice guidelines* (2nd ed., pp. 519–536). St. Louis, MO: Elsevier Saunders.

Black, J., Baharestani, M.M., Cuddigna, J., Dorner, B., Edsberg, L., Langemo, D., et al. (2007). National pressure ulcer advisory panel's updated pressure ulcer staging system. *Advances in Skin and Wound Care, 20,* 269–274.

Edsberg, L. (2007, Winter/Spring). Evidence-based care in pressure ulcer management. *Network Newsletter: An Official Publication of the Association for the Advancement of Wound Care,* p. 9.

Fleck, C.A. (2006). Fighting odor in wounds. *Advances in Skin and Wound Care, 19,* 242–244.

Fulton, J. (2006). Skin metastasis. In D. Camp-Sorrell & R. Hawkins (Eds.), *Clinical manual for the oncology advanced practice nurse* (2nd ed., pp. 139–142). Pittsburgh, PA: Oncology Nursing Society.

Gomez, D., & Policzer, J. (2001). Dermatologic problems. In B. Kinzbrunner, N. Weinreb, & J. Policzer (Eds.), *20 common problems in end-of-life care* (pp. 203–212). New York: McGraw-Hill.

Gupta, S., Bates-Jensen, B., Gabriel, A., Holloway, A., Niezgoda, J., & Wier, D. (2007). Differentiating negative pressure wound therapy devices: An illustrative case series. *Wounds: A Compendium of Clinical Research, 19*(Suppl. 1), 1–9.

Hess, C.T. (2002). *Clinical guide: Wound care* (4th ed.). Springhouse, PA: Springhouse.

Hospice Pharmacia. (2006). *The hospice pharmacia medication use guidelines.* Philadelphia: Author.

Lagman, R., Walsh, D., & Day, K. (2002). Oxidized cellulose dressings for persistent bleeding from a superficial malignant tumor. *American Journal of Hospice and Palliative Care, 19,* 417–418.

Langemo, D., Anderson, J., Hanson, D., Thompson, P., & Hunter, S. (2007). Understanding palliative wound care. *Nursing, 37*(1), 65–66.

Langemo, D., & Brown, G. (2006). Skin fails too: Acute, chronic, and end-stage skin failure. *Advances in Skin and Wound Care, 19,* 206–210.

Mekrut-Barrows, C. (2006). Softening the pain of cancer-related wounds. *Ostomy/Wound Management, 52*(9), 12–13.

Moore, S. (2002). Cutaneous metastatic breast cancer. *Clinical Journal of Oncology Nursing, 6,* 255–259.

Naylor, W. (2002, March). *World wide wounds part I: Symptom control in the management of fungating wounds.* Retrieved July 17, 2007, from http://www.worldwidewounds.com/2002/march/Naylor/Symptom-Control-Fungating-Wounds.html

Niezgoda, J., & Mendez-Eastman, S. (2006). The effective management of pressure ulcers. *Advances in Skin and Wound Care, 19*(Suppl. 1), 3–15.

Pieper, B. (2007). Mechanical forces: Pressure, shear, and friction. In R. Bryant & D. Nix (Eds.), *Acute and chronic wounds: Current management concepts* (3rd ed., pp. 205–230). St. Louis, MO: Mosby.

Queen, D., Woo, K., Schultz, V., & Sibbald, R.G. (2005). Chronic wound pain and palliative cancer care. *Ostomy/Wound Management, 51*(Suppl. 11A), 9–11.

Registered Nurses Association of Ontario. (2002, August). *Assessment and management of stage I to IV pressure ulcers.* Retrieved July 2, 2007, from http://www.guideline.gov/summary/summary .aspx?doc_id=3719&nbr=002945&string=wound+AND+cleansing

Schiech, L. (2002). Malignant cutaneous wounds. *Clinical Journal of Oncology Nursing, 6,* 305–308.

Sharp, C., & McLaws, M. (2005, October). *A discourse on pressure ulcers physiology: The implications of repositioning and staging.* Retrieved July 17, 2007, from http://www.worldwidewounds.com/2005/ october/Sharp/Discourse-On-Pressure-Ulcer-Physiology.html

Warriner, R., & Burrell, R. (2005). Infection and the chronic wound: A focus on silver. *Advances in Skin and Wound Care, 18*(Suppl. 1), 2–11.

Wilson, J., Mills, J., Prather, I., & Dimitrijevich, D. (2005). A toxicity index of skin and wound cleansers used on in vitro fibroblasts and keratinocytes. *Advances in Skin and Wound Care, 18,* 373–377.

Wound, Ostomy and Continence Nurses Society. (2003). *Guideline for prevention and management of pressure ulcers: WOCN clinical practice guideline series, no. 2.* Glenville, IL: Author.

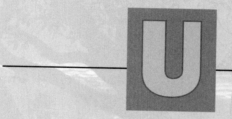

Urinary Elimination

Urinary Elimination

Uthona R. Green, RN, MSN, and Mary E. Murphy, RN, MS, AOCN®, ACHPN

Definition

Urinary elimination is the emptying of urine from the bladder. During the act of urinary elimination, the urine passes from the kidneys down the ureters to the bladder, and then outside the body via the urethra. In males, the proximal urethra is surrounded by the prostate gland. Compared to the male, the female urethra is shorter and in closer proximity to the rectum, thus allowing easier colonization of bacteria, and in turn, leading to a higher prevalence of infection (Jackson, 2007; LeBlond, DeGowin, & Brown, 2004).

Pathophysiology and Etiology

Urinary elimination depends on effective functioning of the primary urinary tract organs: kidneys, ureters, bladder, and urethra. The impairment of any of these organs can produce a variety of disturbing symptoms or life-threatening conditions such as urinary obstruction, renal failure, and urinary incontinence in patients receiving palliative care. Urinary obstruction commonly is caused by gastrointestinal, genitourinary, or gynecologic cancers and most commonly is associated with progressive tumor obstruction of the ureters (Norman & Bailly, 2004). Renal failure usually is secondary to the primary disease process or is associated with side effects from specific medications that are metabolized and excreted by the kidney. The most common causes of an involuntary loss of urine for the patient with advanced malignant disease are direct tumor invasion, surgical intervention, and loss of innervation caused by spinal cord or nerve root damage (Norman & Bailly).

Manifestations

- Decreased or absent urinary output
- Palpable bladder

The authors would like to acknowledge Peg Esper, MSN, MSA, RN, AOCN®, APRN-BC, for her contribution that remains unchanged from the first edition of this textbook.

- Inability or straining to urinate
- Lower abdominal discomfort or pressure
- Hematuria or clots in urine
- Flank or back pain
- Inability to control voiding (leakage)

(Norman & Bailly, 2004)

Management

A. General measures
  1. Identify the underlying cause.
     a) Inability to void
        (1) Obstruction (e.g., tumor, stone, bladder outlet obstruction, clots)
        (2) Oliguria or anuria (e.g., renal failure, when death is imminent)
     b) Involuntary loss of urine
        (1) Prostate cancer (e.g., post-radical prostatectomy, benign prostatic hypertrophy [BPH])
        (2) Neurogenic (e.g., spinal cord compression)
        (3) Genitourinary surgery (e.g., hysterectomy)
        (4) Age-related etiology
        (5) Medication (e.g., sedatives or hypnotics)
     c) Hematuria
  2. Evaluate the need for catheterization.
  3. Evaluate medication profile, and look for possible genitourinary side effects.
  4. Evaluate hydration, and encourage fluid intake where appropriate.
  5. Consider the patient's preferences, adequacy of symptom control, disease progression, and the burden versus the benefit of investigation and intervention (Norman & Bailly, 2004).

B. Death is not imminent.
  1. Obstruction
     a) Pharmacologic interventions
        (1) **Level I—high level of evidence**
            Alpha$_1$ adrenoceptor blocking agent (BPH): Tamsulosin (Flomax®) ($$)—0.4 mg po once daily
        (2) **Level II—moderate level of evidence**
            (a) Antihypertensive BPH (Bruner, Haas, & Gosselin-Acomb, 2005)
                i) Terazosin hydrochloride (Hytrin®) ($)—1 mg po at bedtime
                ii) Doxazosin mesylate (Cardura®) ($)—1 mg po once daily
            (b) Antibiotics for prostatitis (acute or chronic) and prophylactic treatment for indwelling catheters (Nabi, Sheikh, Greene, & Marsh, 2003; Niel-Weise & van den Broek, 2005)

i) Cephalosporins
  - Cefuroxime (Ceftin®) ($$)—750 mg–1.5 g IV every eight hours, usually for 5–10 days
  - Cefotaxime (Claforan®) ($$)—1g IV every 8–12 hours usually for 5–10 days. When the patient has clinically improved, the therapy can be switched to oral treatment according to the patient's sensitivities.
ii) Quinolones
  - Ciprofloxacin (Cipro®) ($$)—500 mg po bid for 28 days
  - Ofloxacin (Floxin®) ($$)—200 mg po bid for 28 days

(3) **Level III—low level of evidence**
  (a) Insertion of 1% alum ($$) irrigation of bladder at a rate of 5 ml/min for a maximum period of 72 hours in continuous bladder irrigation (Moy & Joyce, 2006)
  (b) Synthetic antifibrinolytic agents (aminocaproic acid [Amicar®]) ($$$)—4–5 g in 250 ml IV over the first hour, then 1 g/hour in 50 ml administered continuously for eight hours, or until the bleeding is controlled (Pereira & Phan, 2004)

b) Nonpharmacologic interventions
  (1) **Level I—high level of evidence**
  (Alper & Young, 2006; Cirillo, 2003; Fekete, 2006; Vaglio & Buzio, 2006)
  (a) Percutaneous nephrostomy tubes ($$)—Nephrostomy tubes must be irrigated with 5 ml of bacteriostatic isotonic sodium chloride every 6–12 hours for management.
  (b) Suprapubic catheters ($$)—These catheters lower the risk of bacteriuria and the need for recatheterization and are more comfortable for the patient.
  (c) Dialysis for uremia ($$$)—This intervention should be considered on an individual patient and situation basis and should include patient and family counseling, as well as the identification of anticipated outcomes.

  (2) **Level II—moderate level of evidence**
  (Chung, Stein, Landsittel, Davies, & Cuellar, 2004; Nabi et al., 2003)
  (a) Bladder tumor embolization ($$$)
  (b) Ureteral stents ($$)

  (3) **Level III—low level of evidence**
  (Jamison, Maguire, & McCann, 2007; Moy & Joyce, 2006)
  (a) Intermittent or continuous catheterization ($)
  (b) Continuous or intermittent bladder irrigation ($$) to prevent or treat blood clots

2. Incontinence
  a) Pharmacologic interventions

  (1) **Level I—high level of evidence**
   Antimuscarinics (Scottish Intercollegiate Guidelines Network, 2004)
   (a) Oxybutynin (Ditropan XL®) ($)—5 mg po once daily
   (b) Propiverine (Detrunorm®) ($$)—15 mg po once daily
   (c) Tolterodine (Detrol® LA) ($$)—2 mg po bid
   (d) Trospium (Sanctura®) ($$)—20 mg po once daily, one hour before meal
   (e) Dosage titration should be considered for these medications to reduce adverse effects.
  (2) **Level II—moderate level of evidence**
   Estrogen therapy (Alhasso, Glazener, Pickard, & N'Dow, 2005; Finnish Medical Society Duodecim, 2005; Leach et al., 1997)
   (a) Estradiol (Vagifem®) ($$)—vaginal suppository or tablet once a day at bedtime for two weeks, then three times a week
   (b) Alpha-adrenergic receptor drugs ($)
    i) Doxazosin mesylate—1 mg po once daily
    ii) Pseudoephedrine ($)—15–60 mg po two to three times a day
 b) Nonpharmacologic interventions
  (1) **Level II—moderate level of evidence**
   (Hay-Smith & Dumoulin, 2006; Hunter, Moore, & Glazener, 2007)
   (a) Pelvic floor muscle training ($)—Women are likely to report they have fewer episodes of urinary incontinence with this exercise than do men.
   (b) External penile clamp ($)—Monitoring the patient for safety issues is important.
   (c) External sheath catheters ($)
  (2) **Level III—low level of evidence**
   Disposable pads ($)—Keep skin as dry as possible.

C. Death is imminent.
 1. A gradual decline in the filtering function of the kidneys is a normal occurrence in the dying process.
 2. At this time, comfort is a priority, and use of a Foley catheter may be considered to prevent urinary incontinence that requires frequent bed changes and patient movement.
 3. Evaluate patient and caregiver preferences.

Patient Outcomes

A. Optimal urine elimination is maintained.

B. The incidence of skin breakdown is reduced or prevented.

C. The incidence of infection is reduced.

References

Alhasso, A., Glazener, C., Pickard, R., & N'Dow, J. (2005, May). Adrenergic drugs for urinary incontinence in adults. *Cochrane Database of Systematic Reviews 2003*, Issue 2. Art. No. CD001842. DOI: 10.2002/146518. CD001842.pub2.

Alper, A.B., Jr., & Young, B.A. (2006). *Uremia*. Retrieved May 8, 2007, from http://www.emedicine.com/med/topic2341.htm

Bruner, D.W., Haas, M.L., & Gosselin-Acomb, T.K. (Eds.). (2005). *Manual for radiation oncology nursing practice and education* (3rd ed.). Pittsburgh, PA: Oncology Nursing Society.

Chung, S.Y., Stein, R.J., Landsittel, D., Davies, B.J., & Cuellar, D.C. (2004). 15-year experience with the management of extrinsic ureteral obstruction with indwelling ureteral stents. *Journal of Urology, 172*, 592–595.

Cirillo, R.L., Jr. (2003). *Percutaneous nephrostomy*. Retrieved May 10, 2007, from http://www.emedicine.com/radio/TOPIC796.HTM

Fekete, T. (2006). *Urinary tract infection associated with indwelling bladder catheters*. Retrieved May 10, 2007, from http://www.uptodateonline.com

Finnish Medical Society Duodecim. (2005). *EBM guidelines: Evidence-based medicine*. Helsinki, Finland: Duodecim Medical Publications. Retrieved May 16, 2007, from http://www.guideline.gov

Hay-Smith, E.J.C., & Dumoulin, C. (2006). Pelvic floor muscle training versus no treatment, or inactive control treatments, for urinary incontinence in women. *Cochrane Database of Systematic Reviews 2006*, Issue 1. Art. No.: CD005654. DOI: 10.1002/14651858. CD005654.

Hunter, K.F., Moore, K.N., & Glazener, C.M.A. (2007). Conservative management for post prostatectomy urinary incontinence. *Cochrane Database of Systematic Reviews 1999*, Issue 4. Art. No.: CD001843. DOI: 10.1002/14651858. CD001843.pub3.

Jackson, M.A. (2007). Evidence-based practice for evaluation and management of female urinary tract infection. *Urologic Nursing, 27*, 133–136.

Jamison, J., Maguire, S., & McCann, J. (2007). Catheter policies for management of long term voiding problems in adults with neurogenic bladder disorders. *Cochrane Database of Systematic Reviews 2004*, Issue 2. Art. No.: CD004375. DOI: 10.1002/14651858. CD004375.pub2.

Leach, G.E., Dmochowski, R.R., Appell, R.A., Blaivas, J.G., Hadley, H.R., Luber, K.M., et al. (1997). Female Stress Urinary Incontinence Clinical Guidelines Panel summary report on surgical management of female stress urinary incontinence. The American Urological Association. *Journal of Urology, 158*(3 Pt. 1), 875–880.

LeBlond, R.F., DeGowin, R.L., & Brown, D.D. (2004). *DeGowin's diagnostic examination* (8th ed.). New York: McGraw-Hill.

Moy, B., & Joyce, R.M. (2006). *Cystitis in patients with cancer*. Retrieved May 10, 2007, from http://www.uptodateonline.com

Nabi, G., Sheikh, N., Greene, D., & Marsh, R. (2003). Therapeutic transcatheter arterial embolization in the management of retractable hemorrhage from pelvic urological malignancies: Preliminary experience and long-term follow-up. *British Journal of Urology International, 92*, 245–247.

Niel-Weise, B.S., & van den Broek, P.J. (2005). Antibiotic policies for short-term catheter bladder drainage in adults. *Cochrane Database of Systematic Reviews 2005*, Issue 3. Art. No.: CD005428. DOI: 10.1002/14651858. CD005428.

Norman, R.W., & Bailly, G. (2004). Genitourinary problems in palliative medicine. In D.H. Doyle, G. Hanks, N.I. Cherny, & K. Calman (Eds.), *Oxford textbook of palliative medicine* (3rd ed., pp. 647–657). New York: Oxford University Press.

Pereira, J., & Phan, T. (2004). Management of bleeding in patients with advanced cancer. *Oncologist, 9*, 561–570.

Scottish Intercollegiate Guidelines Network. (2004). *Management of urinary incontinence in primary care: A national clinical guideline*. Edinburgh, Scotland: Author. Retrieved May 14, 2007, from http://www.guidelines.gov

Vaglio, A., & Buzio, C. (2006). *Treatment of retroperitoneal fibrosis*. Retrieved May 10, 2007, from http://www.uptodateonline.com

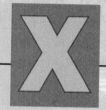

Xerostomia

Xerostomia

LaDonna Hinkle, RN, MSN, OCN®, and
Mary E. Murphy, RN, MS, AOCN®, ACHPN

Definition

Xerostomia is defined as a subjective complaint of mouth dryness caused by decreased saliva production (DeConno, Sbanotto, Ripamonti, & Ventafridda, 2004; Guggenheimer & Moore, 2003). It commonly is seen in patients in the palliative care setting.

Pathophysiology and Etiology

Saliva is produced by the salivary glands and is important in maintaining oral-pharyngeal health. Saliva is essential for lubricating the oral cavity, protecting the mouth from bacterial and fungal infections, preventing dental caries, and aiding in digestion and swallowing (Berk, Shivnani, & Small, 2005; Bruce, 2004). Contributing factors to xerostomia include certain medications (e.g., anticholinergics, tricyclic antidepressants, diuretics, opioids, antihistamines), head and neck irradiation, Sjogren syndrome, dehydration, decreased mastication, poorly controlled diabetes, and head and neck surgery (Bruce; DeConno et al., 2004; Guggenheimer & Moore, 2003). Xerostomia affects eating, drinking, swallowing, and speaking, therefore greatly affecting quality of life.

Manifestations

- Dysphagia
- Dysphonia
- Decreased taste sensation
- Decreased ability to chew
- Mouth soreness
- Thickened or absent saliva

The authors would like to acknowledge Peg Esper, MSN, MSA, RN, AOCN®, APRN-BC, for her contribution that remains unchanged from the first edition of this textbook.

- Cracks or fissures at corner of lips
- Halitosis
- Oral infections

(Bruce, 2004; DeConno et al., 2004; Guggenheimer & Moore, 2003)

Management

Management of xerostomia should focus on providing symptom relief and increasing saliva flow.

A. Death is not imminent.
1. **Level I—high level of evidence**
   Pilocarpine (Salagen®) tablets—($) 5 mg po tid (Aframian et al., 2007; Berk et al., 2005; Haveman, 2004)
2. **Level II—moderate level of evidence**
   (Berk et al., 2005; Bruce, 2004; Jedel, 2005)
   a) Acupuncture ($$)
   b) Cevimeline (Evoxac®) ($$)—30 mg po tid
3. **Level III—low level of evidence**
   (Bruce, 2004; Dirix, Nuyts, & Van den Bogaert, 2006; Guggenheimer & Moore, 2003; Miller & Kearney, 2001; Wiseman, 2006)
   a) Encourage basic oral care.
      (1) The patient should brush teeth with fluoride toothpaste twice a day.
      (2) The patient should floss daily. However, discourage flossing if the patient has a platelet count less than 50,000.
   b) Encourage the patient to rinse with alcohol-free mouth rinses.
   c) Offer the patient sugar-free hard, sour candy and sugar-free chewing gum.
   d) Offer soft, moist foods and add sauces and gravies.
   e) Use artificial saliva products ($) including Biotene® Oral Balance®, Moi-Stir®, and Salivart®.
   f) Use a spray bottle with water to mist the oral cavity.
   g) Apply canola oil to the mouth at bedtime.
   h) Use a humidifier at night.
   i) Use an antifungal agent to treat oral infections, such as nystatin (My-costatin®), or fluconazole (Diflucan®) ($–$$).
   j) Encourage the patient to avoid tobacco, alcohol, carbonated beverages, caffeine, spicy or acidic foods, and sweet hard candies, as they increase dryness and thickness of saliva. Do not use lemon glycerin swabs, as they have a similar effect.

B. Death is imminent.
1. Priority at this time should focus on maintaining the patient's comfort.
2. Provide basic oral care as needed.

Patient Outcomes

A. The oral cavity is adequately lubricated.

B. Optimal comfort is provided.

References

Aframian, D.J., Helcer, M., Livni, D., Robinson, S.D., Markitziu, A., & Nadler, C. (2007). Pilocarpine treatment in a mixed cohort of xerostomic patients. *Oral Diseases, 13,* 88–92.

Berk, L.B., Shivnani, A.T., & Small, W., Jr. (2005). Pathophysiology and management of radiation-induced xerostomia. *Journal of Supportive Oncology, 3,* 191–200.

Bruce, S. (2004). Radiation-induced xerostomia: How dry is your patient? *Clinical Journal of Oncology Nursing, 8,* 61–67.

DeConno, F., Sbanotto, A., Ripamonti, C., & Ventafridda, V. (2004). Mouthcare. In D. Doyle, G. Hanks, N.I. Cherny, & K. Calman (Eds.), *Oxford textbook of palliative medicine* (3rd ed., pp. 673–687). New York: Oxford University Press.

Dirix, P., Nuyts, S., & Van den Bogaert, W. (2006). Radiation-induced xerostomia in patients with head and neck cancer: A literature review. *Cancer, 107,* 2525–2534.

Guggenheimer, J., & Moore, P. (2003). Xerostomia: Etiology, recognition and treatment. *Journal of the American Dental Association, 134,* 61–69.

Haveman, C.W. (2004). Xerostomia management in the head-and-neck radiation patient. *Texas Dental Journal, 121,* 483–497.

Jedel, E. (2005). Acupuncture in xerostomia: A systematic review. *Journal of Oral Rehabilitation, 32,* 392–396.

Miller, M., & Kearney, N. (2001). Oral care for patients with cancer: A review of the literature. *Cancer Nursing, 24,* 241–254.

Wiseman, M. (2006). The treatment of oral problems in the palliative patient. *Journal of the Canadian Dental Association, 72,* 453–458.

Z

Zoster

Zoster (Varicella Zoster Virus—Shingles)

Peg Esper, MSN, MSA, RN, AOCN®, APRN-BC

Definition

Zoster is a viral infection resulting from reactivation of the latent varicella zoster virus (VZV) that lies within the dorsal root ganglia of the spinal cord. Considerable morbidity can result when the virus becomes disseminated outside of its original dermatome. Both cutaneous and visceral dissemination of the virus are possible (Holcomb & Weinberg, 2006).

Pathophysiology and Etiology

Reactivation of VZV is a common complication in terminally ill patients as a result of susceptibility to immunosuppression. The incidence and severity increase with age (Holcomb & Weinberg, 2006; Johnson & Whitton, 2004). Mortality rates as high as 10% have been reported and frequently are linked to the development of VZV pneumonia or central nervous system (CNS) invasion leading to encephalitis (Friel, 2007; Heininger & Seward, 2006; Stone & Hawkins, 2007). Visual complications frequently occur with ophthalmic herpes zoster. Development of postherpetic neuralgia (PHN) is one of the most debilitating complications that occurs from VZV (Volpi, Gross, Hercogova, & Johnson, 2005).

Manifestations

- Vesicular lesions along a dermatome
- Intense neuropathic-like pain
- Abdominal discomfort
- Symptoms related to encephalitis
- Conjunctivitis (ophthalmic VZV)
- Fever

Management

The goal of treatment is to expedite the healing of the rash and to decrease the risk of developing PHN and other complications (Johnson & Whitton, 2004).

A. Death is not imminent.
1. **Level I—high level of evidence**
   Antivirals (Gnann & Whitley, 2002; Lin et al., 2001; Ormrod & Goa, 2000; Sandy, 2005; Shafran et al., 2004; Wood, Kay, Dworkin, Soong, & Whitley, 1996)
   a) Acyclovir (Zovirax®) ($)—800 mg po five times per day for 10 days. This is the least expensive treatment but requires the most frequent dosing.
   b) Famciclovir (Famvir®) ($$)—500 mg po every eight hours for seven days
   c) Valacyclovir (Valtrex®) ($$)—1 g every eight hours for seven days. This medication is more effective in decreasing the risk of PHN than acyclovir.
2. **Level II—moderate level of evidence**
   (Johnson & Whitton, 2004; Wood et al., 1994)
   a) Opioid analgesics ($–$$) (See Pain.)
   b) Topical capsaicin cream ($)—applied four times daily for control of PHN
   c) Corticosteroids ($)—These should not be used in immunocompromised patients or patients with HIV.
   d) Nerve blocks ($$$)
   e) Tricyclic antidepressants ($)—These may decrease development of PHN.
3. **Level III—low level of evidence**
   a) Cold compresses
   b) Meticulous oral care for zoster involving the oral region

B. Death is imminent.
1. Priority is given to maintaining comfort.
2. The use of antivirals during this time is of little value.

Patient Outcomes

A. Symptoms associated with the VZV infection are controlled.

B. The patient's comfort is maintained.

References

Friel, F.J. (2007). Herpes zoster in 2007: Treatment and prevention. *Journal of the American Academy of Physicians Assistants, 20,* 21–25.

Gnann, J.W., Jr., & Whitley, R.J. (2002). Clinical practice: Herpes zoster. *New England Journal of Medicine, 347,* 340–346.

Heininger, U., & Seward, J.F. (2006). Varicella. *Lancet, 368,* 1365–1376.

Holcomb, K., & Weinberg, J.M. (2006). A novel vaccine (Zostavax) to prevent herpes zoster and post-herpetic neuralgia. *Journal of Drugs in Dermatology, 5,* 863–866.

Johnson, R.W., & Whitton, T.L. (2004). Management of herpes zoster (shingles) and postherpetic neuralgia. *Expert Opinion on Pharmacotherapy, 5,* 551–559.

Lin, W.R., Lin, H.H., Lee, S.S., Tsai, H.C., Huang, C.K., Wann, S.R., et al. (2001). Comparative study of the efficacy and safety of valaciclovir versus acyclovir in the treatment of herpes zoster. *Journal of Microbiology, Immunology, and Infection, 34,* 138–142.

Ormrod, D., & Goa, K. (2000). Valaciclovir: A review of its use in the management of herpes zoster. *Drugs, 59,* 1317–1340.

Sandy, M.C. (2005). Herpes zoster: Medical and nursing management. *Clinical Journal of Oncology Nursing, 9,* 443–446.

Shafran, S.D., Tyring, S.K., Ashton, R., Decroix, J., Forszpaniak, C., Wade, A., et al. (2004). Once, twice, or three times daily famciclovir compared with aciclovir for the oral treatment of herpes zoster in immunocompetent adults: A randomized, multicenter, double-blind clinical trial. *Journal of Clinical Virology, 29,* 248–253.

Stone, M.J., & Hawkins, C.P. (2007). A medical overview of encephalitis. *Neuropsychological Rehabilitation, 17,* 429–449.

Volpi, A., Gross, G., Hercogova, J., & Johnson, R.W. (2005). Current management of herpes zoster: The European view. *American Journal of Clinical Dermatology, 6,* 317–325.

Wood, M.J., Johnson, R.W., McKendrick, M.W., Taylor, J., Mandal, B.K., & Crooks, J.A. (1994). A randomized trial of acyclovir for 7 days or 21 days with and without prednisolone for treatment of acute herpes zoster. *New England Journal of Medicine, 330,* 896–900.

Wood, M.J., Kay, R., Dworkin, R.H., Soong, S.J., & Whitley, R.J. (1996). Oral acyclovir therapy accelerates pain resolution in patients with herpes zoster: A meta-analysis of placebo-controlled trials. *Clinical Infectious Diseases, 22,* 341–347.

Appendices

Appendix A
Polypharmacy in Palliative Care

Appendix B
Principles of Pharmacokinetic
Drug Interactions

Appendix C
Internet Resources

Appendix A. Polypharmacy in Palliative Care

Catherine Christen, PharmD

Inappropriate prescribing of medications is a significant cause of morbidity and mortality in the United States and can be particularly problematic with older adults, who often constitute a large portion of the palliative care and supportive care populations. As the number of medications for a patient increases, the risk for prescribing medications that are inappropriate (ineffective, not indicated, or a therapeutic duplicate) increases (Steinman et al., 2006). Patients who take five to six different medications used an average of 0.4 inappropriate drugs, compared to an average of 1.1 inappropriate drugs in patients who take seven to nine different medications, and 1.9 inappropriate drugs in patients taking 10 or more different medications (Steinman et al.). Inappropriate prescribing in older adults with multiple diseases is likely to result in adverse drug reactions, which may result in hospital admissions and further decline in health. Physiologic changes that occur with aging can contribute to alterations in drug pharmacokinetics and pharmacodynamics. A decrease in total body water, hepatic mass, blood flow, renal function, and bone marrow reserve and an increase in body fat occur in older adults as they age. These physiologic changes combined with polypharmacy can be factors in drug interactions and adverse effects (Extermann & Hurria, 2007). Polypharmacy also can result in increased drug expenditures.

The Beers criteria is a common tool used to identify problematic drugs (Fick et al., 2003). The criteria include 48 medications to avoid in older adult patients, including propoxyphene and its combinations, meperidine, amitriptyline, diphenhydramine, long-acting benzodiazepines, muscle relaxants, antispasmodics, and barbiturates (except for anticonvulsant use). Some antihypertensives (clonidine, methyldopa, doxazosin, and guanethidine) are included based on their anticholinergic or sedating adverse effects or risk of orthostatic hypotension or depression. The Beers criteria also list medical conditions and medications that are potentially inappropriate in older adults, which have been extracted in Table 1 (Fick et al.).

When patients opt for comfort or palliative care, only essential medications should be continued (pain medications, antihypertensives, anti-angina agents). Many nonessential medications are discontinued because of drug costs or lack of efficacy, or to reduce the potential for adverse effects. Overlapping adverse drug effects also need to be considered, such as sedation, constipation, and orthostasis,

Table 1. Potentially Inappropriate Medications for Older Adults Based Upon Disease or Condition

Disease or Condition	Drugs	Concern	Severity Rating (High or Low)
Anorexia and malnutrition	CNS stimulants: dextro-amphetamine (Adderall®), methylphenidate (Ritalin®), methamphetamine, and pemoline	Concern because of appetite-sup-pressing effects	High
Arrhythmias	Tricyclic antidepressants (doxepin, imipramine, ami-triptyline)	Concern because of proarrhythmic ef-fects and ability to produce QT interval changes	High
Bladder out-flow obstruc-tion	Anticholinergics, antihis-tamines, antidepressants, decongestants, gastroin-testinal antispasmodics, muscle relaxants, oxybu-tynin (Ditropan®), flavoxate (Urispas®), and tolterodine (Detrol®)	May decrease uri-nary flow, leading to urinary retention	High
Blood clotting disorders or use of antico-agulants	Aspirin, NSAIDs, dipyri-damole (Persantine®), ticlopidine (Ticlid®), and clopidogrel (Plavix®)	May prolong clotting time, elevate INR values, or inhibit platelet aggrega-tion, resulting in increased bleeding potential	High
Chronic con-stipation	Calcium channel block-ers, anticholinergics, and tricyclic antidepressants (imipramine, doxepin, ami-triptyline)	May exacerbate constipation	Low
Cognitive im-pairment	Barbiturates, anticholin-ergics, antispasmodics, muscle relaxants, and CNS stimulants: dex-troamphetamine, meth-ylphenidate, methamphet-amine, and pemoline	Concern because of CNS-altering ef-fects	High

(Continued on next page)

Table 1. Potentially Inappropriate Medications for Older Adults Based Upon Disease or Condition *(Continued)*

Disease or Condition	Drugs	Concern	Severity Rating (High or Low)
COPD	Long-acting benzodiazepines: chlordiazepoxide and combination products (Librium®, Librax®, Limbitrol®), diazepam (Valium®), clorazepate (Tranxene®), and β-blockers	CNS adverse effects. May induce or exacerbate respiratory depression.	High
Depression	Long-term benzodiazepine use. Sympatholytic agents: methyldopa (Aldomet®), reserpine, and guanethidine	May produce or exacerbate depression	High
Gastric or duodenal ulcers	NSAIDs and aspirin (> 325 mg per day). Coxibs excluded.	May exacerbate existing ulcers or produce new ulcers	High
Heart failure	Disopyramide (Norpace®), high-sodium-content drugs	Negative inotropic effect, potential to promote fluid retention	High
Hypertension	Pseudoephedrine, diet products, and amphetamines	May elevate blood pressure because of sympathomimetic activity	High
Insomnia	Decongestants, theophylline, methylphenidate, MAOIs, and amphetamines	Concern because of CNS stimulant effects	High
Obesity	Olanzapine (Zyprexa®)	May stimulate appetite and increase weight gain	Low
Parkinson disease	Metoclopramide (Reglan®), conventional antipsychotics, and tacrine (Cognex®)	Concern because of antidopaminergic or cholinergic effects	High

(Continued on next page)

Table 1. Potentially Inappropriate Medications for Older Adults Based Upon Disease or Condition *(Continued)*

Disease or Condition	Drugs	Concern	Severity Rating (High or Low)
Seizures or epilepsy	Bupropion (Wellbutrin®), clozapine (Clozaril®), chlorpromazine (Thorazine®), thioridazine, and thiothixene (Navane®)	May lower seizure threshold	High
SIADH hyponatremia	SSRIs: fluoxetine (Prozac®), citalopram (Celexa®), fluvoxamine (Luvox®), paroxetine (Paxil®), and sertraline (Zoloft®)	May exacerbate or cause SIADH	Low
Stress incontinence	α-blockers (doxazosin, prazosin, terazosin), anticholinergics, tricyclic antidepressants (doxepin, imipramine, amitriptyline), and long-acting benzodiazepines	May produce polyuria and worsening of incontinence	High
Syncope or falls	Short- to intermediate-acting benzodiazepines and tricyclic antidepressants (imipramine, doxepin, amitriptyline)	May produce ataxia, impaired psychomotor function, syncope, and additional falls	High

CNS—central nervous system; COPD—chronic obstructive pulmonary disease; INR—international normalized ratio; MAOIs—monoamine oxidase inhibitors; NSAIDs—nonsteroidal anti-inflammatory drugs; SIADH—syndrome of inappropriate antidiuretic hormone secretion; SSRIs—selective serotonin reuptake inhibitors

Note. From "Updating the Beers Criteria for Potentially Inappropriate Medication Use in Older Adults: Results of a U.S. Consensus Panel of Experts," by D.M. Fick, J.W. Cooper, W.E Wade, J.L. Waller, J.P. Maclean, and M.D. Beers, 2003, *Archives of Internal Medicine, 163,* pp. 2719–2721. Copyright 2003 by the American Medical Association. Adapted with permission.

and this criterion can be useful in removing unneeded drugs from the medication profile. Additionally, medications to consider discontinuing in palliative care patients include those that are not indicated, have a long time frame for therapeutic benefit, or are therapeutic duplicates (e.g., two different benzodiazepines), or medications with long duration of activity in the setting where death is imminent. Examples of medications that should be considered for discontinuation in patients receiving palliative care are listed in Table 2.

Table 2. Examples of Medications That Can Be Discontinued in Patients Managed With Palliative Care

Medication	Rationale
Amiodarone	Discontinue with imminent death because of long plasma half-life.
Amitriptyline	Anticholinergic effects, sedation
Amphetamines (excluding methylphenidate)	CNS stimulant adverse effects
Aspirin	Discontinue if used for secondary prevention
Barbiturates (except for anticonvulsant use)	Sedation, respiratory depression
Bisphosphonates	Time frame for therapeutic benefit
Colony-stimulating factors (epoetin, darbepoetin, filgrastim)	Time frame for therapeutic benefit
Cyclandelate, isoxsuprine	Lack of efficacy
Diphenhydramine	Sedation
Estrogens	Carcinogenic potential and lack of cardioprotective effects in older women
Ethacrynic acid	May cause fluid imbalances
Fluoxetine	Long duration of action, risk of sleep disturbances and agitation (because of excessive CNS stimulation)
Guanethidine, guanadrel, doxazosin, short-acting nifedipine, clonidine	May cause orthostasis
Herbal or complementary and alternative medications	Lack of evidence of benefit, potential cost savings for the patient
Iron supplements	Time frame for therapeutic benefit
Long-acting benzodiazepines: flurazepam, diazepam, clorazepate, chlordiazepoxide	Sedation, respiratory depression
Long-term use of full-dose non-COX-selective NSAIDs with long durations of action: naproxen, oxaprozin, piroxicam	Potential for gastrointestinal bleeding, renal failure, high blood pressure, and heart failure

(Continued on next page)

Table 2. Examples of Medications That Can Be Discontinued in Patients Managed With Palliative Care *(Continued)*

Medication	Rationale
Long-term use of stimulant laxatives, except with opioid use: bisacodyl, cascara	May exacerbate bowel dysfunction
Methyltestosterone	Potential for prostatic hypertrophy and cardiac problems
Mineral oil	Potential for aspiration
Nitrofurantoin	Potential for renal impairment
Opioids (some): propoxyphene, meperidine	Lack of efficacy and many disadvantages compared to other opioids
Orphenadrine	Sedation and anticholinergic effects
Proton pump inhibitors, H_2 antagonists	Exception: patients with current symptomatic gastritis or reflux esophagitis avoid cimetidine because of CNS effects.
Statins	Time frame for cardiovascular disease because of high cholesterol levels
Thioridazine, mesoridazine	CNS and extrapyramidal effects
Ticlopidine	Adverse effects; not shown to be better than aspirin
Vitamin supplements	Time frame for therapeutic benefit

CNS—central nervous system; COX—cyclooxygenase; NSAIDs—nonsteroidal anti-inflammatory drugs

Note. Based on information from Currow et al., 2007; Fick et al., 2003.

References

Currow, D.C., Stevenson, J.P., Abernethy, A.P., Plummer, J., & Shelby-James, T.M. (2007). Prescribing in palliative care as death approaches. *Journal of the American Geriatrics Society, 55,* 590–595.

Extermann, M., & Hurria, A. (2007). Comprehensive geriatric assessment for older patients with cancer. *Journal of Clinical Oncology, 25,* 1824–1831.

Fick, D.M., Cooper, J.W., Wade, W.E., Waller, J.L., Maclean, J.R., & Beers, M.D. (2003). Updating the Beers criteria for potentially inappropriate medication use in older adults: Results of a U.S. consensus panel of experts. *Archives of Internal Medicine, 163,* 2716–2724.

Steinman, M.A., Landefeld, C.S., Rosenthal, G.E., Berthenthal, D., Sen, S., & Kaboli, P.J. (2006). Polypharmacy and prescribing quality in older people. *Journal of the American Geriatrics Society, 54,* 1516–1523.

Appendix B. Principles of Pharmacokinetic Drug Interactions

David Frame, PharmD

Many drug-drug interactions are likely to be encountered while caring for palliative care patients. Drug-disease and drug-food interactions may occur as well, which make prescribing medications even more challenging. Basic pharmacokinetic principles can be useful in recognizing and avoiding drug-drug interactions in the management of palliative care patients.

Pharmacokinetic interactions occur when the action of one drug alters the serum concentration of another drug through changes in absorption, distribution, metabolism, or excretion (King, 2003). For example, a more alkaline gastric pH from the use of H_2-blockers or proton pump inhibitors may decrease absorption of itraconazole, ketoconazole, or indinavir. Often, cachexia and increased catabolism cause a decrease in albumin, to which many drugs bind. This decrease in albumin may result in higher levels of free drug in the system, which may increase the distribution of the drug, as well as the proportion of active drug in the body, thus resulting in not only increased efficacy but also increased toxicity (Baker & Parton, 2007).

Many drugs are substrates for and are metabolized by the cytochrome P450 system. One of the greatest risks of drug interactions is caused by changes in enzymatic clearance. Some drugs, such as phenytoin or rifampin, may induce or increase cytochrome P450 enzyme activity, which can decrease the levels of the drugs that are substrates for a particular enzyme, thus resulting in decreased efficacy (Gorski et al., 2003). However, some agents, such as voriconazole, itraconazole, posaconazole, or cimetidine, are inhibitors of certain P450 enzymes and could increase the level of other substrates of those enzymes, which could result in increased toxicity (Saad, DePestel, & Carver, 2006). The greatest concentrations of these enzymes are in the liver; however, these enzymes are also in the gastrointestinal tract, which often results in more interaction when drugs are given orally than when administered intravenously. Figure 1 includes agents that are substrates for the different enzymes in the cytochrome P450 system. These drugs may have their clearance reduced when given with substances that inhibit those enzymes (see Figure 2) or may have their clearance increased when given with substances that induce these enzymes (see Figure 3).

In addition to pharmacokinetic interactions, pharmacodynamic interactions may also occur where drugs may have synergistic, additive, or antagonistic effects that may cause changes in drug efficacy and/or toxicity (King, 2003).

Figure 1. Drugs That Are Substrates to the Cytochrome P450 System

CYP 1A2
- Acetaminophen
- Amitriptyline
- Caffeine
- Clomipramine
- Clozapine
- Cycloben-
  zaprine
- Estradiol
- Fluvoxamine
- Haloperidol
- Imipramine
- Naproxen
- Olanzapine
- Ondansetron
- Propanolol
- Theophylline
- Verapamil
- Warfarin
- Zileuton
- Zolmitriptan

CYP 2B6
- Bupropion
- Cyclophos-
  phamide
- Efavirenz
- Ifosfamide
- Methadone

CYP 2C8
- Cerivastatin
- Paclitaxel
- Repaglinide
- Torsemide

CYP 2C19
- Amitriptyline
- Citalopram
- Clomipramine
- Cyclophos-
  phamide
- Diazepam
- Imipramine
- Indomethacin
- Lansoprazole
- Nelfanivir
- Omeprazole
- Pantoprazole
- Phenytoin
- Phenobarbital
- Primidone
- Progesterone
- Propanolol
- Teniposide
- Warfarin

CYP 2C9
- Amitriptyline
- Celecoxib
- Diclofenac
- Fluoxetine
- Fluvastatin
- Glyburide
- Glipizide
- Glimeparide
- Irbesartan
- Ibuprofen
- Losartan
- Naproxen
- Phenytoin
- Rosiglitazone
- Tamoxifen
- Warfarin

CYP 2D6
- Carvedilol
- Chlorfen-
  iramine
- Chlorprom-
  azine
- Clomipramine
- Codeine
- Debrisoquine
- Desipramine
- Dextromethor-
  phan
- Encainide
- Flecainide
- Fluoxetine
- Haloperidol
- Imipramine
- Lidocaine
- Metoclopra-
  mide
- Metoprolol
- Mexiletine
- Nortriptyline
- Ondansetron
- Oxycodone
- Posaconazole
- Promethazine
- Propanolol
- Resperidol
- Tamoxifen
- Tramadol
- Venlafaxine

CYP 2E1
- Ethanol
- Theophylline

CYP 3A4,5,7
- Alprazolam
- Amlodipine
- Aprepitant
- Atorvastatin
- Buspirone
- Caffeine
- Chlopheniramine
- Clarithromycin
- Codeine
- Cyclosporine
- Dapsone
- Dasatinib
- Dexamethasone
- Dextromethorphan
- Diazepam
- Diltiazem
- Erythromycin
- Estradiol
- Felodipine
- Fentanyl
- Granisetron
- Hydrocortisone
- Imatinib
- Haloperidol
- Lidocaine
- Lovastatin
- Methadone
- Midazolam
- Nifedipine
- Ondansetron
- Progesterone
- Propanolol
- Quinine
- Resperidol
- Simvastatin
- Sirolimus
- Tacrolimus
- Tamoxifen
- Testosterone
- Trazodone
- Verapamil
- Zolpidem

Note. Based on information compiled from www.micromedex.com.

Figure 2. Cytochrome P450 Inhibitors

CYP 1A2
- Amiodarone
- Cimetidine
- Fluoroquino-
  lones

CYP 2B6
- Ticlopidine

CYP 2C8
- Glitazones
- Gemfibrozil
- Montelukast
- Trimethoprim

CYP 2C19
- Chloramphenicol
- Cimetidine
- Fluoxetine
- Indomethacin
- Ketoconazole
- Voriconazole
- Lansoprazole
- Omeprazole
- Probenecid
- Ticlopidine
- Topiramate

CYP 2C9
- Amiodarone
- Fluconazole
- Fluvastatin
- Isoniazid
- Lovastatin
- Probenecid
- Sertraline
- Sulfamethox-
  azole
- Voriconazole

CYP 2D6
- Amiodarone
- Bupropion
- Celecoxib
- Chlorprom-
  azine
- Chlorphen-
  iramine
- Cimetidine
- Citalopram
- Clomipramine
- Diphenhydra-
  mine
- Duloxetine
- Fluoxetine
- Haloperidol
- Hydroxyzine
- Metoclopra-
  mide
- Methadone
- Midodrine
- Paroxetine
- Quinidine
- Ritonavir
- Sertraline

CYP 2E1
- Disulfiram

CYP 3A4,5,7
- Amiodarone
- Aprepitant
- Cimetidine
- Clarithromycin
- Dasatinib
- Diltiazem
- Erythromycin
- Fluconazole
- Fluvoxamine
- Grapefruit juice
- Imatinib
- Itraconazole
- Ketoconazole
- Norfloxacin
- Posaconazole
- Verapamil
- Voriconazole

Note. Based on information compiled from www.micromedex.com.

Figure 3. Cytochrome P450 Inducers

CYP 1A2
- Broccoli
- Brussels
  sprouts
- Insulin
- Nafcillin
- Omeprazole

CYP 2B6
- Phenobarbital
- Rifampin

CYP 2C8
- Rifampin

CYP 2C19
- Carbamazepine
- Prednisone
- Rifampin

CYP 2C9
- Rifampin

CYP 2D6
- Dexametha-
  sone
- Rifampin

CYP 2E1
- Ethanol
- Isoniazid

CYP 3A4,5,7
- Barbiturates
- Carbamazepine
- Efavirenz
- Glucocorticoids
- Phenobarbital
- Phenytoin
- Rifampin
- St. John's wort
- Troglitazone
- Rifabutin

Note. Based on information compiled from www.micromedex.com.

Drug-Disease Interactions

Drug interactions can arise as a result of pharmacokinetic changes caused by symptoms of the patient's disease. Absorption of foods and drugs often is compromised because of changes in the gastrointestinal system. Diarrhea generally results in decreased absorption of drugs because of decreased transit time. However, significant constipation may increase absorption, which can be especially problematic with long-acting agents, such as sustained-release opioids. Patients with hepatic disease also may have a change in enzymatic levels, such as decreased albumin and increased bilirubin, which can affect drugs that pass through the P450, glucuronidation, and other hepatic pathways. Changes in the renal elimination of drugs also occur with advancing disease and can be especially important for renally cleared agents.

Food-Drug Interactions

Food may interfere with drug activity in several ways. Of course, the potential exists to either increase or decrease absorption when a drug is administered with food. The product information should always be checked to see if food makes a difference with absorption. Sometimes drugs in the same class may even have very different effects when given with food. For example, itraconazole needs an acidic environment for best absorption; voriconazole absorbs better on an empty stomach; and posaconazole requires not only a meal but preferably one with a high fat content for adequate absorption. Some foods are fortified with vitamins and minerals that can interact with certain drugs, and taking large doses of vitamins can also interfere with some drugs (see Table 1).

Table 1. Food-Drug Interactions

Agent	Mechanism	Potentially Affected Drugs
Calcium • Milk • Dairy products • Fortified orange juice	Absorption	Decreased absorption of • Quinolones • Tetracyclines • Bisphosphonates • Cefuroxime • Methotrexate
Grapefruit juice	Inhibit cytochrome P450 3A4	See Figure 2 for CYP 3A4 inhibitors. Special considerations: • Calcium channel blockers • Tricyclic antidepressants • Benzodiazepines • Amiodarone • Calcineurin inhibitors

(Continued on next page)

Table 1. Food-Drug Interactions *(Continued)*

Agent	Mechanism	Potentially Affected Drugs
High-protein food	Absorption	Increased absorption of • Propanolol Decreased absorption of • Carbidopa • Levodopa • Theophylline
High-fiber food	Absorption	Decreased absorption of • Metformin • Levothyroxine • Digoxin • Penicillin
Vitamin K • Green leafy vegetables	Inhibits vitamin K-dependent epoxide	Increases the effect of warfarin

Note. Based on information from Hulisz & Jakad, 2007.

References

Baker, M., & Parton, T. (2007). Kinetic determinants of hepatic clearance: Plasma protein binding and hepatic uptake. *Xenobiotica, 37,* 1110–1134.

Gorski, J.C., Vannaprasaht, S., Hamman, M.A., Ambrosius, W.T., Bruce, M.A., Haehner-Daniels, B., et al. (2003). The effect of age, sex, and rifampin administration on intestinal and hepatic cytochrome P450 3A activity. *Clinical Pharmacology and Therapeutics 74,* 275–287.

Hulisz, D., & Jakad, J. (2007). Food-drug interactions: Which ones really matter? *U.S. Pharmacist, 32,* 93–98.

King, R. (2003). Drug interactions in the cancer chemotherapy patient. In B. Furie & P. Cassileth (Eds.), *Clinical hematology and oncology: Presentation, diagnosis, and treatment* (pp. 534–556). Philadelphia: Elsevier.

Saad, A.H., DePestel, D.D., & Carver, P.L. (2006). Factors influencing the magnitude and clinical significance of drug interactions between azole antifungals and select immunosuppressants. *Pharmacotherapy, 26,* 1730–1744.

Appendix C.
Internet Resources

Kim K. Kuebler, MN, RN, APRN-BC

Palliative and End-of-Life Care Resources

- American Academy of Hospice and Palliative Medicine
  www.aahpm.org
- Center to Advance Palliative Care
  www.capc.org
- EPERC: End of Life/Palliative Education Resource Center
  www.eperc.mcw.edu
- Growth House
  www.growthhouse.org
- Harvard Medical School Center for Palliative Care
  www.hms.harvard.edu/cdi/pallcare/pcep.htm
- International Hospice and Palliative Care Association
  www.hospicecare.com
- National Comprehensive Cancer Network Palliative Care Guidelines
  www.nccn.org
- National Consensus Project for Quality Palliative Care
  www.nationalconsensusproject.org
- National Hospice and Palliative Care Organization
  www.nhpco.org
- Palliative Care Policy Center
  www.medicaring.org
- Promoting Excellence in End-of-Life Care
  www.promotingexcellence.org
- Regional Palliative Care Program, Edmonton, Alberta, Canada
  www.palliative.org
- San Diego Hospice and Palliative Care
  www.sdhospice.org
- World Health Organization
  www.who.int/cancer/palliative/definition/en

Pain Management Resources

- American Geriatrics Society
  www.americangeriatrics.org
- American Pain Society and the American Academy of Pain Medicine
  www.ampainsoc.org
- American Society of Addiction Medicine
  www.asam.org
- International Association for the Study of Pain
  www.iasp-pain.org
- Dannemiller Memorial Educational Foundation Pain.com
  www.pain.com

Nursing Resources

- Hospice and Palliative Nurses Association
  www.hpna.org
- Oncology Nursing Society
  www.ons.org

Caregiver Resources

- Caring Connections
  www.caringinfo.org
- End-of-Life Choices: CPR and DNR Fact Sheet
  www.caregiver.org/caregiver/jsp/content_node.jsp?nodeid=397
- Family Caregiver Alliance/National Center on Caregiving
  www.caregiver.org
- Spousal Caregiver Support
  www.wellspouse.org

Index

Index

D

L

lactulose (Chronulac®), for constipation, 72
lansoprazole (Prevacid®), for cough, 79
laser therapy, for mucositis, 189
laxatives, 72–73
    discontinuation in palliative care, 276*t*
    for pain, 207
leukotriene modifiers, for cough, 77
Levels of Evidence schema, xvi
levofloxacin (Levaquin®), for cough, 78
levomepromazine
    for bowel obstruction, 196
    for nausea and vomiting, 196
lidocaine (Lidoderm®), for pruritus, 225–227
living will, definition of, 3
local anesthetics, for pruritus, 226
loperamide (Imodium®), for diarrhea, 112
loratadine (Claritin®), for pruritus, 226
lorazepam (Ativan®)
    for anxiety, 31–32
    for delirium, 102
    for palliative sedation, 220
    for seizures, 233
loss. *See* grief
Lubriderm®, for pruritus, 226
lymph drainage, manual, 181
lymphedema, 179–183
    definition of, 179
    management of, 180–181
    manifestations of, 180
    pathophysiology/etiology of, 179

M

malignant cutaneous wounds
    definition of, 241
    management of, 242–247
    manifestations of, 242
    pathophysiology/etiology of, 241
    staging of, 243
malnutrition, inappropriate medications for, 272*t*
manipulative methods, definition of, 62*t*
manual lymph drainage, for lymphedema, 181
MAOIs. *See* monoamine oxidase inhibitors
massage
    contraindications to, 243
    for fatigue, 134
    for lymphedema, 181
    for pain, 209
Medicaid Waiver Program, 57
medications
    during dying process, 92–93
    interactions of, 277–281, 278*t*–279*t*

interactions with disease, 280
interactions with food, 280, 280*t*–281*t*
polypharmacy, 271–276
potentially inappropriate in older adults, 272*t*–274*t*
that can be discontinued in palliative care, 275*t*–276*t*
megestrol acetate, for cachexia, 16
meperidine, discontinuation in palliative care, 276*t*
mesoridazine, discontinuation in palliative care, 276*t*
Metamucil®, for diarrhea, 113
methadone
    for pain, 207
    for pruritus, 225
methamphetamine, contraindications to, 272*t*
methyldopa (Aldomet®), contraindications to, 273*t*
methylphenidate (Ritalin®)
    contraindications to, 272*t*–273*t*
    for depression, 107
    for fatigue, 133
    for hiccups, 161
methylprednisolone (Medrol®), for dyspnea, 120
methyltestosterone (Android®)
    discontinuation in palliative care, 276*t*
    for pruritus, 225
metoclopramide (Reglan®)
    for bowel obstruction, 50
    for cachexia, 18
    contraindications to, 273*t*
    for hiccups, 161
    for nausea and vomiting, 196*t*
metoproterenol (Alupent®), for dyspnea, 119
metronidazole (MetroGel®), for skin lesions, 246
micronutrient deficiencies, enteral feeding and, 21
midazolam
    for delirium, 102
    for dyspnea, 120
    for hiccups, 161
    for palliative sedation, 220
    for seizures, 233
milk of magnesia, for constipation, 72
mind-body interventions, definition of, 62*t*
mineral oil, discontinuation in palliative care, 276*t*
mirtazapine (Remeron®)
    for anxiety, 32
    for pruritus, 226
mistletoe, for fatigue, 134